Keto Diet Cookbook

2 Books in 1: Over 100 Low-Carb, High Fat Keto Recipes on a Budget to Lose Weight, Heal Your Body and Reset Your Metabolism Quick and Easy

Audrey Lane

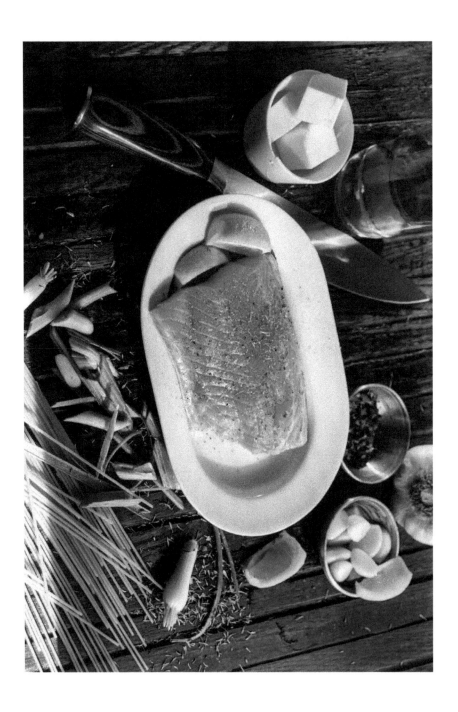

THIS BOOK INCLUDES:

BOOK 1:

The Keto Diet:

The Complete Guide to Ketogenic Diet for Beginners. Easy and Tasty Keto Recipes to Lose Weight, Burn Fat, Balance Hormones, Heal Your Body and Regain Confidence

BOOK 2:

Keto Diet for Beginners Cookbook:

From Breakfast to Dessert, Many Tasty Keto Recipes to Reset Your Metabolism, Lose Weight and Improve Your Health without Losing the Pleasure of Food

The Keto Diet

The Complete Guide to Ketogenic Diet for Beginners. Easy and Tasty Keto Recipes to Lose Weight, Burn Fat, Balance Hormones, Heal Your Body and Regain Confidence

Audrey Lane

Table of Contents

Introduction

What the ketogenic diet does is shock the body into a heightened metabolism by dropping carbohydrates and replacing them with healthy fats. In doing this, your body will be forced to find other sources of energy rather than that which is drawn from consuming carbs.

This process ends up being ketosis. Simply, this refers to the phenomenon when fats are the most significant source of nutrients that your body converts into energy.

This energy emerges from the fat cells that have accumulated within your body. In this way, it is not strictly the foods you eat that contribute to your body's energy. Ketosis thrives off of the fat and energy that already exists within your body. This process is integral for jacking up your metabolism and making it easier to lose weight.

Breakfast Recipes

Bacon and Eggs

We will start this section with one of the most basic and classic breakfast recipes there is. Notably, there are no carbohydrates like home fries or toast added to this dish, which you might find at any given restaurant's take on this recipe. Still, this dish is very filling and a quick and easy fix to start your three-week program.

Ingredients
- Bacon (four strips)
- Eggs (two)
- Salt (for seasoning)
- Pepper (for seasoning)

Cooking Instructions:
Take any amount of bacon slices that you think you will want for this meal.

A recommended number is four slices along with your eggs, but feel free to play with these numbers. Just ensure that you do not add too much or starve yourself.

Take your bacon slices and heat them over the stove at a moderate to high temperature.

Let it cook to your liking (soft or crispy) and then plate them.

Then put the eggs in the pan and prepare them in whatever fashion you like. For this recipe we recommend cooking one side and keeping them covered so that the yolk can cook through.

You can also cook both sides uncovered, flipping when it is beginning to harden. The recipe is as simple as that. Add salt and pepper as seasonings and enjoy!

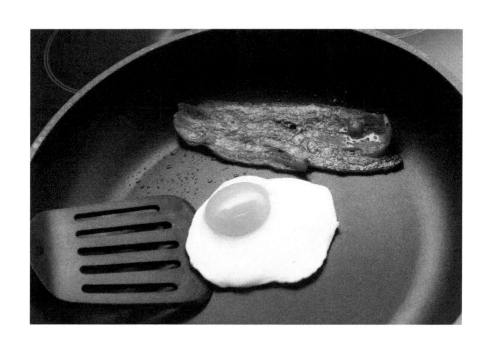

Spinach Frittata

This is another filling and savory recipe. It incorporates spinach and bacon above an egg base as its main ingredients, ensuring that you are getting a healthy helping of vegetables along with your fats and proteins.

Ingredients

- Bacon (four strips)
- Eggs (four)
- Shredded cheese (two ounces)
- Heavy cream (one-half cup)
- Spinach (four ounces)

Cooking Instructions:

In an oven, set your heat to three hundred fifty Fahrenheit. Find a square dish for baking and make sure it is greased.

Like the last recipe, heat your bacon at a moderately high temperature to whatever consistency you prefer.

Before it has concluded cooking, add the spinach so that it can fully cook down. Let these contents cool when they are done.

Take your eggs and combine them with the heavy cream. When they are fully mixed, pour them into the dish that you have chosen for baking.

Put the bacon and spinach that you have already cooked and spread them on top of the layer of eggs, also adding the shredded cheese to the top layer.

Leave this in the oven for about twenty-five minutes, a half-hour tops.

It should have darkened to a very light brown. Cut up into squares and serve on a plate once it has cooled enough to eat.

Coconut Porridge

Here, we switch from savory to a more sweet and dense volume of breakfast. This is a simple meal that requires little preparation and should make your transition into keto eating very easy.

Ingredients

- Shredded coconut (one cup)
- Coconut milk (two cps.)
- Water (two and a half cps.)
- Coconut flour (one-quarter cup)
- Cinnamon (one-half tsp.)
- Nutmeg (one-quarter tsp.)
- Vanilla extract (one tsp.)

Cooking Instructions:

Take your shredded coconut and place it in a small saucepan on the stove at a moderate to hot temperature.

Heat it up until it is toasted, but do not let it sit for too long or the flavor may go from nutty to more burnt.

Once the coconut has reached this point, place the coconut milk and water along with what you have cooked in the pan.

Get these ingredients covered and let them heat up to the point that they are boiling.

When the mixture has reached the point of boiling, take it off of the stove. Add the coconut flour, vanilla extract, cinnamon, and nutmeg.

Take a spoon and mix everything together to the point that it is very well combined. Scoop a healthy portion into a bowl and enjoy!

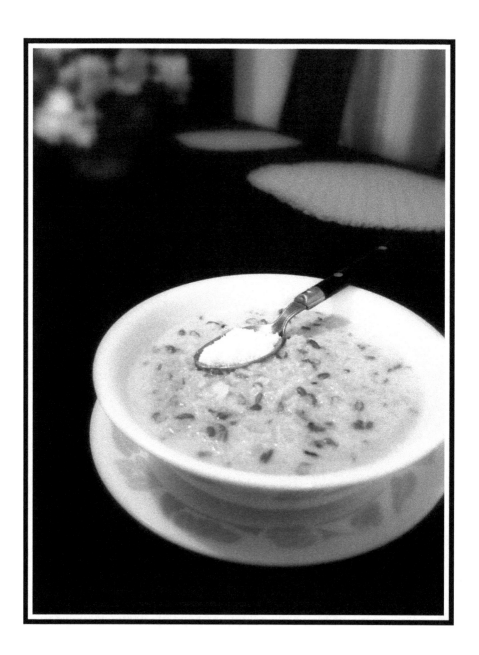

Pancakes

Here, we have a healthy and low carb take on what is typically a breakfast that is very high in carbohydrates.

The trick to this dish is that it uses almond flour as a base rather than a classic pancake mix.

While this recipe is a twist on a dish that is a classic staple of breakfast, it is no less delicious, and it remains a convenient and quick option.

Ingredients
- Almond flour (one-half cup)
- Baking powder (one-half tsp.)
- Salt (one pinch)
- Egg (one)
- Almond milk (one-quarter cup)
- Avocado oil (one Tbsp.)
- Vanilla extract (one-half tsp.)

Cooking Instructions:

This recipe requires heavy mixing of many of the ingredients that are on the shopping list.

Take your almond flour, baking powder, salt, one egg, almond milk, avocado oil, and vanilla extract and place them all in a large bowl.

The next step is as easy as mixing all of this together until they are consistent, and any chunks or clumps in the batter are smoothed out.

Next, put a griddle on the stove and get the temperature up to a moderate level of heat.

You can decide how big you want your pancakes to be, so simply scoop the batter onto the stove at the sizes of pancakes that you desire and repeat the process until your batter is gone.

Breakfast-Style Pizza

This is one of the most unique breakfast recipes in the whole book.

A pizza is inherently designed for a crowd of people, so cooking this may leave you with a heap of leftovers, but there is nothing wrong with that.

Another way around that is taking the serving size of this pizza and simply bringing the ingredients down to a smaller quantity.

This pizza serves anywhere from four to eight people since it is easier to cook that way. If you are dedicated to creating no leftovers for this program, then divide everything in this recipe by about four and you should get the yield of a one-person meal.

Servings aside, this is a very fun and adventurous breakfast. One does not usually picture pizza as a breakfast food, but once you see the variety of ingredients and how they are used, it will become clear that this may be your new favorite way to start the day.

Ingredients

- Eggs (twelve)
- Heavy cream (one-half cup)
- Sausage (eight ounces)
- Chopped bell peppers (two cps.)
- Shredded cheese (one cup)
- Salt (for seasoning)
- Pepper (for seasoning)

Cooking Instructions:

Set your cooking heat to three hundred fifty. To prepare for this dish, get all of the ingredients out.

Microwave your chopped peppers for several minutes so that they are hot enough to cook with the rest of the ingredients.

Put your chopped bits of sausage in a pan/skillet on the stove and let it heat for a couple of minutes to the point that it becomes slightly browned.

Then, remove the sausage and put them on a plate or cutting board off the side.

Next, take the eggs, heavy cream, pepper, and salt. and put them in the pan/skillet.

These ingredients should cook for a few minutes until the egg starts to form and solidify on the edges.

Then, take the pan/skillet (which must be oven safe) and put it in the oven. If you cook it for about ten minutes, you will come out with a softer crust.

Fifteen minutes is the maximum that you should let it cook and that will result in a crunchy crust.

When that time is up, remove these contents and add the sausage and cheese.

Then broil everything for an additional three minutes or so. Once that time is up, remove the contents and let them cool for several minutes so that the pizza is not too hot to handle.

Use a pie cutter to retrieve slices. Refrigerate whatever you do not eat if you chose to make the family-sized portion. Enjoy!

Waffles

Like pancakes, waffles are thought of as a breakfast that is very high in carbohydrates.

This dish takes similar steps to cut down the carb content for the sake of the keto macronutrient guidelines.

As a meal itself, these waffles are fun and simple (which is why they are scheduled for a Sunday morning on your meal plan).

Ingredients
- Egg (one)
- Almond flour (one-half cup)
- Baking powder (one-half tsp.)
- Salt (one pinch)
- Almond butter (two Tbsps.)
- Butter (two Tbsps.)
- Almond milk (one-quarter cup)
- Vanilla extract (one-half tsp.)

Cooking Instructions:

To get the perfect texture for these waffles, it is a bit more complicated than simply throwing some eggs into a bowl with mix and combining it.

First, you must let your waffle iron heat up. Of course, if you do not own a waffle iron it is not necessary to use this dish for your meal plan.

Simply substitute it for something else. But if you do own an iron, make sure it is plugged in and heating as you prepare. Once it has come to a moderate temperature, spray it with oil for non-stick.

Take your egg and crack it so that only the white ends up in a bowl while the yolk still rests in its shell.

Use a whisk or an electric eggbeater to whip up these whites until they stiffen. In a different bowl, mix the almond flour, salt, and baking powder.

Take your almond butter and normal butter and put them together in the microwave. Make sure they are fully melted, then make sure that they are mixed well.

Next, put the butter with the almond flour, salt, and baking powder. In addition, place the yolk of the egg, the almond milk, and vanilla extract to the bowl.

Stir all of this together to the point that it has significantly smoothened. Add the whites that you have whipped and mix that well.

The result should be creamy and light in texture.

Now you are ready to get the batter cooked. Simply place a healthy helping into your waffle iron until all of the surface is covered.

Make sure not to overfill as that will result and leakage, but also be careful not to underfill because that will result in overcooked and thin waffles.

Cooking usually takes three to five minutes. Usually, the presence of steam indicates that the waffles are done.

Once all of the batter has been cooked, plate the waffles. Be careful with toppings like fruit or honey as they are high in carbs. Enjoy!

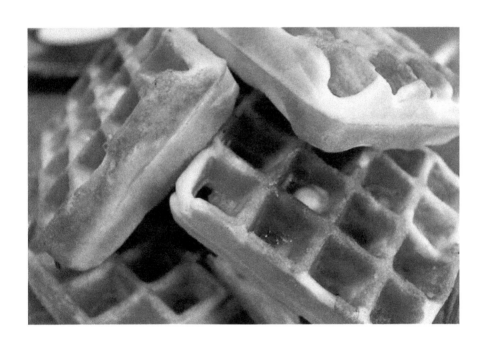

Biscuits

Biscuits are another breakfast food that is synonymous with carbohydrates and conjure up images of sweet, bready dishes.

Where the pancake and waffle recipes use almond flour as a base, these biscuits use coconut flour which is similarly bereft of carbs and can be used for seemingly starchy dishes.

These biscuits are more savory than sweet, but they still have an interesting mix of flavors that makes for a delicious breakfast.

Ingredients
- Butter (one Tbsp.)
- Coconut flour (two Tbsps.)
- Baking powder (one-quarter tsp.)
- Onion powder (one-eighth of a tsp.)
- Garlic powder (one-eighth of a tsp.)
- Salt. (one-eighth of a tsp.)
- Pepper (one-eighth of a tsp.)
- Parsley (one eight of a tsp.)
- Egg (one)
- Shredded cheddar cheese (one-quarter cup)
- Heavy cream. (one Tbsp.)

Cooking Instructions:

Take your butter and put it in a bowl. Microwave it for about thirty seconds until it has fully melted.

Add coconut flour, baking powder, onion powder, garlic powder, salt, pepper, and parsley.

Mix everything up until it is combined with the melted butter.

Next, insert one egg, cheddar cheese, and heavy cream.

Make sure everything is well combined to the point that it is one creamy and thick consistency.

Move this mixture into a receptacle like a mug that will hold its shape well.

Then, microwave the mixture for upwards of three minutes. Because of the nature of the mixture, this will be enough for it to harden into a soft instant biscuit.

Scoop out with a knife and enjoy!

Steak and Eggs

This version of steak and eggs skirts the expectation of being alongside toast and home fries.

Rather, this is essentially a veggie bowl topped with steak and eggs.

It is another easy recipe but one that looks and tastes great when you have finished preparing it.

Ingredients

- Olive oil (one-quarter cup)
- Dijon mustard (one Tbsp.)
- Worcestershire sauce (two Tbsps.)
- Flank steak (one and half pounds)
- Eggs (three)
- Heavy cream (one Tbsp.)
- Avocado (one)
- Salt (for seasoning)
- Pepper (for seasoning)

Cooking Instructions:

Start by taking the olive oil, Dijon mustard, and Worcestershire sauce and mixing them all together in a bowl, as they will serve as the marinade for the meat.

Take the steak and let it rest in the marinade for about an hour. When that process has concluded, give it a final glaze on both sides.

Since this is a breakfast meal, it is recommended that you marinate your steak overnight so that you can enjoy it ready to go in the morning.

The next step is to get a pan/skillet that is resistant to sticking. Get the stove to a moderate to high temperature and place the steak over the heat, cooking for about four to five minutes on both sides.

Do not leave it on too long or it will blacken, but of course be aware of cooking it enough to ensure that it is not too rare.

When this is done, put the steak on a plate or cutting board, also removing the pan/skillet from the heat.

Take your eggs and vigorously mix them with the heavy cream. Once it is well combined, you can cook the eggs.

Retrieve the pan/skillet that you have removed from the heat, first ensuring that it has cooled down enough for another use. You should wipe it down to get the last of the steak off.

Then scramble your eggs at a moderate to low temperature until they reach the texture that you prefer. For creamier, less hardened eggs, cook for a shorter time.

The final few steps of this recipe consist of putting the bowl together. Put the eggs in a bowl as the bottom layer. Then cut your steak into slices.

About four half-inch cuts should be perfect for the dish. Place these slices on top of the eggs. Next, take half an avocado and cut it up into a few slices, placing them on top of the steak.

Season everything with salt and pepper and enjoy your protein-packed breakfast!

Homemade Bagels

While this meal requires you to make something from scratch, it also requires only five ingredients.

These bagels look and taste like your favorite carb-loaded breakfast, but they consist of a handful of far less detrimental ingredients.

You will be the foremost observer of this as you are making these bagels from the ground up.

Ingredients
- Almond flour (one-half cup)
- Baking (one-third Tbsp.)
- Mozzarella cheese (one cup)
- Cream cheese (one ounce)

Cooking Instructions:

First, set your oven's heat to four hundred degrees. Take your almond flour and put it in a bowl with the baking powder.

Stir these ingredients together until they are well combined. Next, take your mozzarella cheese along with the cream cheese and put them together into a bowl.

Throw this bowl in the microwave for no more than three minutes. When the cheeses are done heating, they should be very soft, but they should not be liquidized as butter becomes in the microwave. Stir them to ensure that they are perfectly mixed.

The following aspects of this recipe are time-sensitive so you must perform these tasks consecutively without taking too much time in between.

Take an egg and the mixture of flower and baking powder and throw them into the bowl with the cheeses. Use your hands to mix everything together and knead the substance which will become increasingly doughier.

Remove it from the bowl and place it onto a cutting board when it becomes substantive enough.

If the dough is a bit too difficult to handle, you can place it in the microwave for anywhere from ten to twenty seconds.

This will make it softer and make the kneading process easier. Once you are done with the kneading, everything should be completely combined and of one consistency.

There should be no chunks or bits that stick out.

You are making two bagels with this amount of dough so divide what you have just kneaded into two separate piles on the cutting board.

Separately, roll each of them into long cylindrical shapes. They will eventually be folded into the shape of a bagel, so envision this when you are performing this step.

They should be roughly an inch in diameter and not too long that they will not come together for a bagel of normal size.

When the long cylindrical shapes are formed, wrap them around so that one end meets the other.

You will have two bagel shapes from the dough. Retrieve a pan for baking and cover it with paper for cooking.

Let the bagels cook for anywhere from ten to fifteen minutes.

They should have darkened in color and they should look significantly hardened without having any kind of crunch.

Remove the bagels from the oven and let them cool before consuming with some cream cheese if you like!

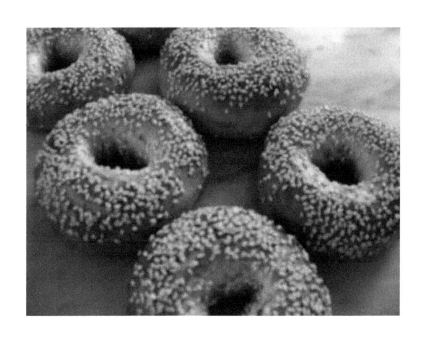

Breakfast Burrito

The breakfast burrito is a deceptively simple way to make breakfast. It includes all of our favorite high fat, low carb centerpieces and comes together for a brilliant ensemble of flavor that you are guaranteed to love.

Ingredients

- Shredded mozzarella cheese (three-quarter cps.)
- Shredded cheddar cheese (one-quarter cup)
- Eggs (two)
- Chives (one-half tsp.)
- Bacon (three strips)

Cooking Instructions:

To make this burrito keto, you need to make your own tortilla. The first step toward doing this is putting a pan/skillet over a moderate temperature.

Once it has heated, add the shredded mozzarella and make sure that it is spread as evenly as possible. The idea is to get this cheese into a hardened and clear shape.

When you see that the edges of the cheese are getting especially crisp, take it off the stove (it should be the shape of a tortilla) and put it on a plate to the side.

Separately, take the shredded cheddar cheese and put it in a bowl with the eggs and chives. Whisk all of this together until it is consistent and include salt and pepper as seasonings.

At this point, cook the bacon on the stove, as demonstrated in previous recipes, and microwave two to three of your frozen breakfast sausages or heat them separately on the stove as well.

Take a new pan/skillet and put one small slice of butter on until it has melted into a non-stick substance. Place the eggs onto the stove at a moderate temperature and scramble them to your liking.

The final step is assembling the burrito. Lay your cheese tortilla down flat on a plate. Place the sausage down first on the tortilla first, then add the eggs, and finally add the bacon as the final layer.

To finish the burrito, fold two of the edges inward and roll the rest of it up. Your keto burrito is ready to eat!

French Toast

French toast is another dish that is synonymous with sweet and relatively unhealthy ways of eating breakfast.

This delicious keto creation, however, is not only formed from coconut flour and some of our favorite sources of fat and protein, but it is also one of the simplest recipes in this book.

Ingredients
- Butter (two Tbsps.)
- Heavy cream (two tsps. and an additional Tbsp.)
- Eggs (two)
- Baking powder (one-half tsp.)
- Coconut flour (two Tbsps.)
- Cinnamon (one-quarter tsp.)
- Vanilla extract (one-half tsp.)

Cooking Instructions:

Take the butter and two tsps. of heavy cream, along with one egg, baking powder, and coconut flour and put all of these ingredients into a bowl.

Whisk everything together to the point that it is consistent. Then, put this dish in the microwave for about a minute and half. This should allow all of the contents to cook.

Once this mixture is out of the microwave, it will resemble a bread. Cut it into slices and set it aside.

Separately, take one egg, the cinnamon, vanilla extract, and the one Tbsp. of heavy cream.

Whisk all of these together until they make the coating for the French toast.

Set a pan/skillet on the stove at a moderate temperature. While it is heating, dip the slices of bread into the coating so that they are covered on both sides.

When the stove has reached the proper heat, fry your slices of bread on both sides until they become golden brown. Enjoy!

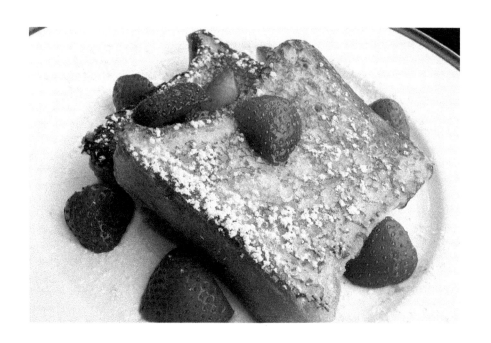

Appetizers and Snacks Recipes

Cheese Crisps

This recipe takes cheese and uses it as the centerpiece for a replacement to a classic chip.

Because chips are obviously too high in carbohydrates to be included in the keto diet, these substitutes add flavor and flair while staying high in fats and protein.

Ingredients
- Grated cheese (six Tbsps.)
- Provolone cheese slices (two)
- Jalapeño pepper (one)

Cooking Instructions:

Set your oven's heat to four hundred twenty-five degrees.

Get a sheet for baking and make sure it is covered in parchment paper or any other non-stick layer that is safe for the oven.

Set your grated cheese into six separate small piles across the pan. Slice up the jalapeño into six different portions.

Place one on each of the small piles of cheese. Cook these contents for roughly five minutes.

Remove these from the oven and use your hands to split the provolone into six smaller pieces total. Cover each mound of grated cheese and jalapeños with some of the provolone.

Put all of this back in the oven for eight to ten minutes until everything has become crisp and brown. They should have a solid crunch to them.

Remove them from the oven, let them cool slightly and enjoy with a low-carb dipping sauce of your choice.

Pizza Bites

This falls more in the category of appetizer than snack in the sense that it is a perfect crowd-pleaser for a group or party.

It removes the bread from the equation and instead uses meats and cheeses as the primary ingredients for a pizza dish.

Ingredients

- Pepperoni (twelve slices)
- Basil leaves (twelve)
- Mozzarella balls (twelve)
- Pizza sauce

Cooking Instructions:

Set your oven's heat to four hundred degrees.

Take your slices of pepperoni and make small cuts at either end so that if you measured a straight line across the diameter, the cuts would both be ends of the line.

This is to make it easier to fit the pepperoni into a muffin pan. This muffin pan should be designed for mini muffins and/or cupcakes.

Place each slice of pepperoni into a mold on a twelve-piece muffin pan.

Put this into the oven for about five minutes. This will allow the pepperoni to get crispy but not overcooked.

Take the pepperoni out of the muffin pan once they are cool enough and put them on a paper towel where they can be drained of grease.

When that process has finished, put each piece of pepperoni back into the muffin pan.

Also add one basil leaf, about one-half tsp. of sauce, and a mozzarella ball per mold.

Put these contents back into the oven for an additional two minutes or so.

The cheese should be melted, and each position should look like a small pizza by itself. Let the contents cool and enjoy!

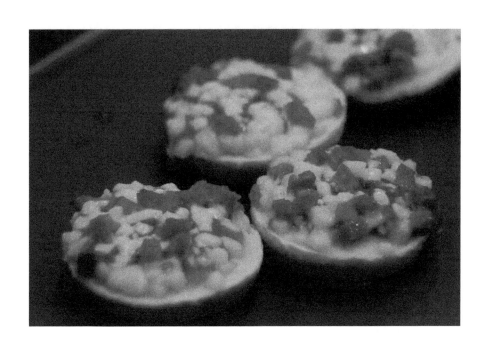

Egg Salad Bites

This is a very interesting dish that, as you will see, features an eclectic mix of flavors and food types. This is within the deviled egg family while also being in the salad family.

Ingredients

- Two hard-boiled eggs
- Four tomatoes (small)
- One and three-quarter Tbsps. of mayonnaise
- Two strips of bacon
- One-half tsp. of chives
- A pinch of paprika

Cooking Instructions

After you have boiled your eggs, cut them up with a fork and lightly mash them so that they are significantly softened but not wholly flattened.

In a bowl, put these eggs with the mayonnaise, also adding pinches of salt and pepper for flavor. Mix these contents together until they are consistent and well-incorporated.

Get your four tomatoes and slice off the tops. Hollow the whole thing out so that it resembles a bowl shape.

Take your egg mixture and scoop it into the tomatoes one at a time. Each of the four tomatoes should be full of heaping scoops so that a bit of the egg is popping out of the top.

The next step is optional, but if you feel inclined, fry some bacon as demonstrated in earlier recipes.

Then break this bacon up into bits and sprinkle some on top of each of the eggs.

This can add some salty flavor and delicious fat to the dish. In addition, top everything with chives and paprika and enjoy!

Popcorn Chicken

This is a contagiously fun recipe. It turns chicken into the type of finger food that can be mass consumed, all while doing so with a fun and easy recipe.

Ingredients

- Chicken breast (one-half pound)
- Buttermilk (three-quarter cps.)
- Chili powder (one-half tsp.)
- Almond flour (one-quarter cup)
- Almonds (one-quarter cup)
- Olive oil
- Lemon juice (from about half a lemon)
- One-quarter cup of mayonnaise
- One-quarter tsp. of chipotle powder
- One-eighth tsp. of garlic powder
- One-half tsp. of tomato paste

Cooking Instructions:

Set your oven's heat to four hundred twenty-five degrees. Take your chicken breast and cut it up into cubes that are about an inch thick, then top it with the chili powder in a bowl.

Next, add your buttermilk, get the bowl covered and refrigerate it for several hours or overnight.

Meanwhile, put the almond flour and almonds into a processor pulse it until it becomes flakey. Put these contents into a separate bowl.

When the chicken is ready to finish marinating, take it out of the bowl and press it into the almond powders, which essentially act as breading.

Put the chicken bits onto a sheet that is safe for baking, but first make sure it is greased with a small layer of olive oil.

Let the chicken cook for roughly fifteen minutes. It should be a nice shade of brown and look crispy to the bite. While it cooks, prepare your dipping sauce.

All you have to do for this step is to put the lemon juice, mayonnaise, chipotle powder, garlic powder, and tomato paste into a bowl.

Mix these well and make sure that all of the colors have meshed, and the texture is consistent along with the shade of the sauce.

At this point, the chicken is probably ready to be removed from the oven.

Let the dish cool for several minutes, then enjoy them on a platter with the dipping sauce that you have just prepared.

Since this is made for a group, store the ones you do not eat, or make sure that you have company when you prepare it.

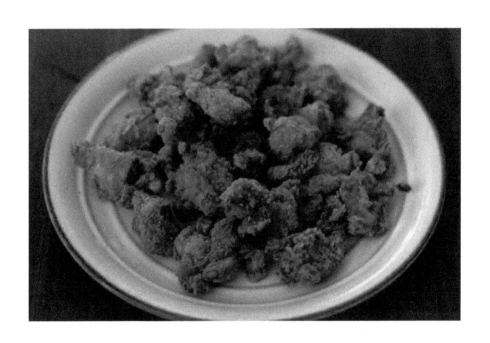

Kale Chips

This is the easiest and healthy a recipe can get. You will be able to tell from the recipe that this meal requires almost no preparation and it yields a fun and simple snack.

Ingredients

- Kale (one bunch)
- Olive oil (one-half Tbsp.)

Cooking Instructions:

Set your oven's heat to four hundred degrees. Take the kale and put it in a bowl after removing all of the stems and ribs.

Then top the kale with your half Tbsp. of olive oil as well as pinches of salt and pepper for taste. Using your hands or a pair of tongs, mix all of this up until each leaf of kale is well covered in oil.

Put the kale onto a pan for cooking. They will not stick because they are oiled. Put the pan in the oven for about five minutes.

The kale should be crisp and have a good snap and crunch to it. Let them cool and enjoy!

Fish and Poultry Recipes

Shrimp and Vegetable Salad

The first meal in this section presents a fun mix of seafood and vegetables. Shrimp is a favorite of many eaters, even those who do not particularly like fish. In this dish, it is the centerpiece of a light and flavorful salad.

Ingredients

- Shrimp (four ounces)
- Butter (one Tbsp.)
- Avocado (one-half – sliced)
- Tomato (one-half – sliced)
- Feta crumbles (one-quarter cup)
- Lemon juice (one-half Tbsp.)
- Olive oil (one-half Tbsp.)
- Cilantro (one pinch)
- Salt (one pinch)
- Pepper (one pinch)
- Parsley (one pinch)

Cooking Instructions:

Take your shrimp along with the butter which you have melted in the microwave for thirty seconds (see other recipes).

Mix these together until the shrimp has been well coated. Put a pan/skillet over a moderate to high temperature. Put the shrimp in and let it cook for about thirty seconds to a minute on both sides.

They should begin to look pink in addition to cooking through the middle.

When the shrimp are done, put them on a plate and allow their temperature to cool.

Take all your remaining ingredients and throw them all into a bowl.
Mix everything together gently so that there are no areas that are too concentrated in any one ingredient.

Take the shrimp from the plate and add it to the salad. You are all set to enjoy this delicious and light meal.

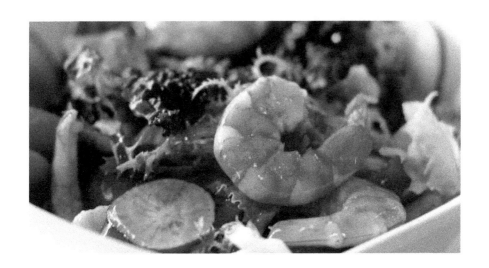

Garlic Chicken

This is a basic chicken recipe that uses a classic simple combination of chicken and garlic to achieve a stunningly vibrant flavor.

Ingredients

- Olive oil (one and half Tbsps.)
- Chicken breast (one)
- Heavy cream (one cup)
- Chicken broth (one-half cup)
- Italian seasoning (one tsp.)
- Garlic powder (one tsp.)
- Parmesan cheese (one-half cup)
- Spinach (one cup)
- Sundried tomatoes (one-half cup)

Cooking Instructions:

Add the olive oil to a pan/skillet over a moderate temperature on the stove. Let each side of the chicken breast cook for about four minutes until the skin has browned and the center is no longer pink.

This is very important not only for the taste and texture of the chicken but also for safety's sake. Once you have cooked your chicken, remove it from the stove and put it on a plate to use later in the recipe.

Take a bowl and add the heavy cream, chicken broth, Italian seasoning, garlic powder, and parmesan.

Put all of this into another pan/skillet at a higher temperature this time. Whisk the ingredients while they heat to the point that the liquid becomes thicker.

At this point, add your spinach and sundried tomatoes. Once the spinach is wilting, you can put the chicken in with the rest of the ingredients until everything is warm and ready to serve!

Chicken Salad

Chicken salad is a great recipe to have around because it is very versatile in how it can be used. It's perfect as a standalone meal but it can also be used as a side for leftovers or even as a dip for cheese crisps.

You can get adventurous with this meal and the upcoming recipe gives you a clear and full look at how to make it the best way possible.

Ingredients

- Bacon (six strips)
- Chicken breast (one)
- Avocado (one)
- Sliced celery (one-quarter cup)
- Scallions (one-quarter cup)
- Cheddar cheese (one-quarter cup)
- Salt (one pinch)
- Pepper (one pinch)
- Dressing (one-half cup)

Cooking Instructions:

First, take the bacon and fry it over the stove like you have in many previous recipes in this book. Put them onto a towel for drainage and once most of the grease has been absorbed, chop the bacon up into little bits.

To cook the chicken, leave a small bit of the bacon fat in whatever pan/skillet you have just used. Add the chicken breast and cook it for about ten minutes on both sides, covering the pan with a lid both times.

When the chicken is done being cooked, take it off of the heat and let it cool down for several minutes. When it has sufficiently cooled down, cut it up into cubes that can be used for the salad.

In a large bowl, throw in the avocado that you have sliced up into small cubes, along with the sliced celery, scallions, and cheddar cheese.

Then add the pinches of salt and pepper along with some dressing. Throw the cubes of chicken in and mix everything together so that the dressing is layered and combined into the texture. Enjoy immediately or stick in the fridge until you are ready to serve.

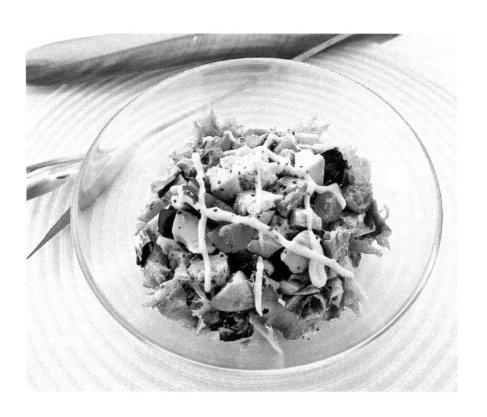

Salmon

Salmon is the healthiest fish there is. It is also one of the more pristine sources of seafood, which makes it a perfect ingredient to form a meal around.

This dish is a frittata of sorts, but nothing draws more attention in flavor or in nutrition than the salmon itself.

Keep in mind that this is a large dish that is made for a group so be sure to keep your consumption to one or two servings.

Ingredients

- Heavy cream (one-half cup)
- Eggs (eight)
- Salt (one pinch)
- Pepper (one pinch)
- Onion (one – chopped)
- Smoked salmon (four ounces)
- Zucchini (one – sliced)
- Parsley (two Tbsps.)
- Chives (two Tbsps.)
- Chopped dill (four Tbsps.)

Cooking Instructions:

Set your oven's heat to three hundred fifty degrees. Take the heavy cream along with eggs and salt and pepper and whisk everything together until it is combined and still notably creamy.

Retrieve a pan/skillet that is also safe for oven use. Put it on the stove at a moderate temperature and add the slices from the chopped onion. Sauté for a few minutes until the onion is see-through and the flavors are pungent.

Take the stove's heat down to moderate and throw in the smoked salmon, zucchini, parsley and chives, chopped dill, and a bit of salt and pepper for taste.

Then take the mixture of eggs and cream that you made at the beginning of the recipe and douse all of the other ingredients in the pan.

Cook everything for about six or so minutes until the cream begins to stiffen and can be removed from the pan.

Take everything off of the stove and put it in the oven (in the oven-safe pan/skillet).

Let the contents cook for anywhere from fifteen to twenty minutes. You will know it is done when there is no more flimsiness to the center.

Remove the pan from the oven, let it cool for several minutes, then cut yourself a piece and enjoy!

Chicken Fajitas

This is another dish that is flashy and has a lot of moving parts but really just serves as a showcase for the chicken at the center of it all.

You can't go wrong with chicken as it is a protein source that includes healthy fats, while also working with an extreme variety of flavors.

Ingredients:
- Chili powder (one tsp.)
- Paprika (one-half tsp.)
- Garlic powder (one-half tsp.)
- Cumin (one-half tsp.)
- Salt (one pinch)
- Pepper (one pinch)
- Cayenne (one pinch)
- Chicken breast (one)
- Lime juice (from one lime)
- Olive oil (two Tbsps.)
- Bell peppers (two)
- Onion (one-half)

Cooking Instructions:

Set your oven's heat to four hundred degrees. Take the chili powder, paprika, garlic powder, and cumin, along with pinches, of salt, pepper, and cayenne.

Put all of these contents into a mason jar. Shake the jar thoroughly until all of the spices have mixed.

Next, put your chicken breast into a sealable plastic bag. Juice a lime into the bag and add half of the olive oil.

Then take the seasoning that you have just made and add about two to three tsps. Seal the bag tightly and lightly press down on the chicken so that it absorbs all of the flavor.

If you choose, simply seal the bag and refrigerate it overnight. This will allow the chicken to fully marinate in the seasonings.

Take the bell pepper and onion and slice them up, eventually placing them on a pan that will go in the oven.

Put the rest of the olive oil on these vegetables and make sure that they are coated.

When the chicken is ready, put that on the pan next to, but not on top of the peppers and onion.

Put these contents in the oven for about nine minutes, at which point you should take it out, turn the chicken over, and gives the vegetables a mix.

Then, put it back in the oven and cook for an additional ten or so minutes, or until the chicken has cooked through the middle and to a pleasant brown on the outside.

If the chicken is taking too long, remove the vegetables from the oven first so that they don't burn while the chicken is cooking.

Remove the contents from the oven and let them cool to a reasonable temperature.

Since this is keto, do not use any tortillas to wrap them with. Instead use sliced avocados as a topping and eat the dish with a fork.

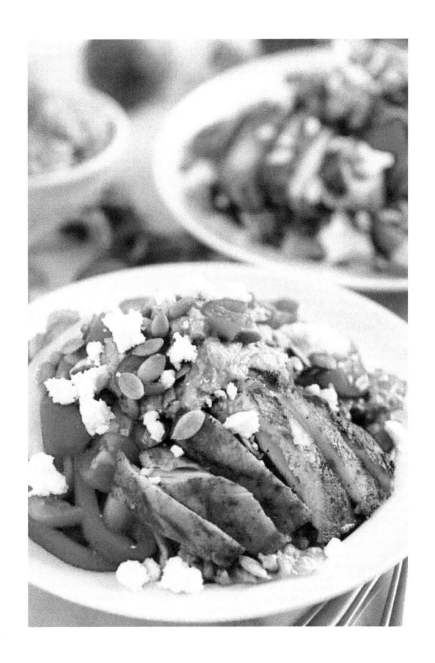

Chicken Enchilada

Like the previous recipe, this dish uses chicken with a bit of a twist. It creates an enchilada in a very loose sense of the word.

Like the fajitas, there are no tortillas used as they are too high in carbs.

Instead, this dish uses zucchini as the base, creating a delicate and delicious vegetable-packed version of an enchilada.

Ingredients
- Zucchini (two)
- Olive oil (one Tbsp.)
- Ground chicken (one-half pound)
- Taco seasoning (two Tbsps.)
- Cream cheese (two ounces)
- Sour cream (one-quarter cup)
- Green verde sauce (one-half cup)
- Shredded cheese (one-half cup)

Cooking Instructions:

Set your oven's heat to three hundred fifty degrees. Get a deep pan that is made for casseroles and dishes of that nature, drizzling it with olive oil.

Take your zucchinis and slice them into halves the long way so that you have four vertical zucchini halves. Take a spoon and remove the middle of the zucchini, hollowing it out so that the chicken filling can go in.

Once you are done with this, place the zucchinis into the pan with the hollow sides facing up. Drizzle them with the olive oil and season lightly.

Put foil onto the zucchini and put it in the oven. It should cook for about twenty-five minutes.

Meanwhile, take a skillet/pan and put it over a moderate to high temperature. Add olive oil for greasing, then put the ground chicken on.

Cook it in full until it is browned and cooked through. Next, add the store-bought taco seasoning of your choice (with flavor and macros in mind) with a dash of water.

Mix all of this together until the chicken has been coated. Then, do the same with the cream cheese, sour cream, green verde sauce, and shredded cheese of your choice.

When you are done mixing all of these ingredients, make sure they are covered if the zucchini is still cooking.

When the twenty-five minutes are up, take the zucchini out of the oven and spoon the mixture evenly into each hollowed-out vegetable.

Then, cover with additional shredded cheese (just enough for a nice melted layer) and put everything back in the oven for fifteen to twenty minutes.

Remove the contents when they are done, let them cool, and enjoy!

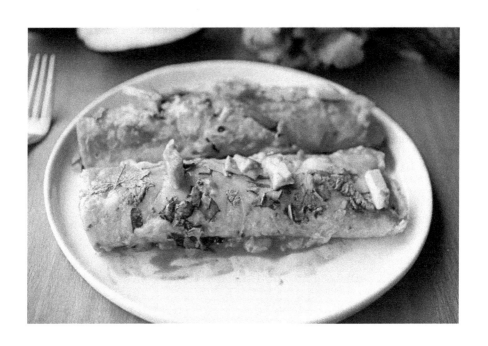

Meats Recipes

Sloppy Joe

This first recipe is a dinner dish that subs out the normal carbs of the buns for lettuce. It's a particularly rich and hearty option that is perfect as a dinner for someone who is craving a lot of flavor.

It uses a slow cooker, so be sure to start preparing this meal hours in advance of whatever time you plan to eat it.

Ingredients
- Ground beef (two pounds)
- Pork sausage (one pound)
- Onion (one – diced)
- Garlic (three cloves – minced)
- Tomato sauce (eight ounces)
- Tomato sauce (two Tbsps.)
- Apple cider vinegar (two Tbsps.)
- Sugar-free ketchup (three-quarter cps.)
- Chili powder (one Tbsp.)
- Worcestershire sauce (one Tbsp.)

- Mustard (three Tbsps.)
- Salt (for seasoning)
- Romaine lettuce (a few large leaves)

Cooking Instructions:

Retrieve a pan/skillet and put it over a moderate to high temperature. Add ground beef, pork sausage, and the onion. Let this all cook until the onion has significantly softened, which should be anywhere from five to ten minutes.

Retrieve a crockpot and spray it down with canola oil or any other spray of your choice that will prevent sticking. Place the contents from the pan inside.

Add the garlic, about tomato sauce, tomato paste, apple cider vinegar, sugar-free ketchup, chili powder, Worcestershire sauce, mustard, and some salt to bring out the flavor.

Give the whole pot a mix so that everything combines, then turn to pot onto a low setting for about five hours.

It is as simple as that. You will know it's done when the sloppy joe has reached the right consistency of soft but not too runny.

Get a large leaf of romaine lettuce and add some heaping scoops to enjoy your carb-free sloppy joe.

Curry Meatballs

This is technically a chicken recipe, but because of the connotation of "meatball," we will put it in the meat section. These meatballs are doused in flavor and consist of tenderly packed chicken. This is a very involving recipe that consists of a handful of ingredients and flavors.

Ingredients

Side Salad:
- Cabbage (four cps.)
- Vinegar (two Tbsps.)
- Honey (one-half Tbsp.)
- Cilantro (one-quarter cup)
- Lemon juice (from one lemon)
- Salt (for seasoning)
- Pepper (for seasoning)

Main Course:
- Ground chicken (one pound)
- Chili powder (one Tbsp.)
- Basil (one Tbsp.)
- Olive oil (one Tbsp.)
- Cumin (one Tbsp.)

- Garlic powder (one-half Tbsp.)
- Chili paste (one-half Tbsp.)
- Egg (one)
- Flour (one-quarter cup)
- Rolled oats (one-quarter cup)
- Salt (one pinch)

Curry Sauce:

- Olive oil (one Tbsp.)
- Onion (one – sliced)
- Garlic (one clove – minced)
- Coconut milk (one can)
- Red curry paste (three Tbsps.)
- Hot sauce (one Tbsp.)
- Lime juice (three Tbsps.)

Cooking Instructions:

Set your oven's heat to four hundred degrees. Get a large dish for cooking that is made for casseroles and grease it with canola oil or coconut oil.

Separately, get a large bowl and toss in cabbage (purple or green), vinegar, honey, cilantro, lemon juice, and salt and pepper for seasoning. Mix all of these ingredients up and put them in the fridge.

This will be your side salad.

The next step is to form the meatballs. Take all of the ingredients from the Main Course section and mix these together as the material that you will scoop your meatballs out of.

To do this, take an ice cream scooper and scoop out as many meatballs as you can from the meatball mix. Put them all into the pan that you prepared earlier. Let them cook in the oven for about ten minutes.

While the meatballs are in the oven, you will make your curry sauce. Put a pan/skillet on the stove at a moderate to high temperature. Throw the olive oil in and add some onion once it is hot enough.
Let this cook for about two minutes then throw in the minced garlic, coconut milk, red curry paste, hot sauce of your choice, and lime juice and cook at the highest setting for about two more minutes.

When the meatballs have been in the oven for ten minutes, remove them to add the sauce evenly. Let all of this cook for another eight or so minutes.
Remove from the oven, take the side cabbage out of the fridge and serve everything together.

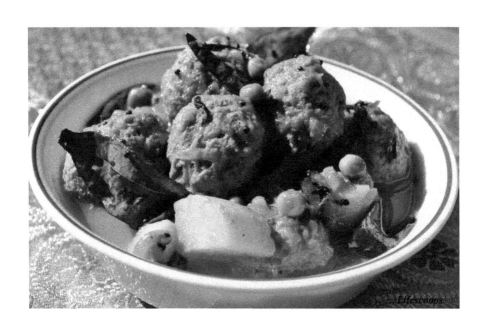

Sausage and Peppers

This regional favorite presents a great way to fulfill your craving for a hot dog or any kind of similarly unhealthy meaty meal. This, however, is a much healthier option, bursting with vegetables and flavor to boot. The recipe is also incredibly simple and easy to pull off.

Ingredients

- Olive (one Tbsp. and an additional three Tbsps.)
- Kielbasa (twelve ounces - sliced)
- Bell peppers (four – sliced)
- Pepper (for seasoning)

Cooking Instructions:

Take a pan/skillet and put it over the stove at a moderate temperature. Add a Tbsp. of olive oil to grease the pan along with the sliced kielbasa.

Let this cook for several minutes until they go from pink to pinkish-brown and look and taste smoky. When it is done, take the kielbasa off of the pan.

Put another three Tbsps. of olive oil onto your pan/skillet along with the bell peppers (any color or mix of colors for these bell peppers will work).

Heat the peppers for several minutes until they become soft and tender.

Then, put the sausage back into the pan to get them back to a warm temperature.

Add pepper and whatever other spices you may have a taste for.

Cook for about one minute then remove the ingredients from the heat and serve with sour cream.

Pork Chops

These pork chops present a very singular recipe. The pork, which is a very rich and succulent meat, is the center of the meal with very few frills are things to take away from it besides a garlic sauce that only adds layers to the flavors and texture.

Ingredients

- Olive oil (two tsps.)
- Pork chops (three – boneless)
- Pepper (for seasoning)
- Paprika (one tsp.)
- Butter (two Tbsps.)
- Garlic (six cloves – minced)
- Onion (one – minced)
- Italian seasoning (one tsp.)
- Red pepper flakes (one tsp.)
- Chicken stock (one-third of a cup)
- Heavy cream (one and a half cps.)
- Spinach (three cps.)
- Shredded parmesan cheese (one-quarter cup)
- Parsley (one pinch)

Cooking Instructions:

To start, take the olive oil and put it on a pan/skillet at a moderate to high temperature.

Take the pork chops and distribute some pepper and paprika on both sides of each piece of pork.

Place them all into the pan and let them cook for about four minutes on each side until they have browned, and the middles are cooked.

When these are done cooking, you can take them off of the heat and put them on a plate to be used later.

Put the butter into the same pan and then add the garlic, one onion, Italian seasoning and red pepper flakes.

Let everything cook for a few minutes until it is very fragrant. Next, add the chicken stock and cook until it starts to reduce.

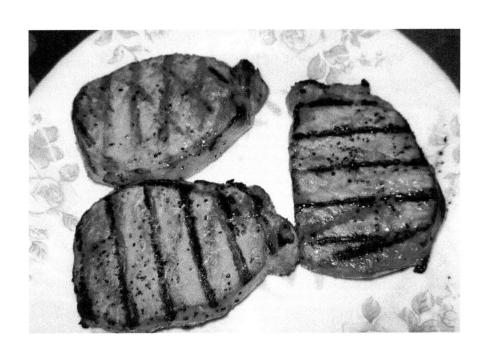

Veggies and Sides Recipes

Zucchini Pasta

While pasta is synonymous with carbohydrates, one common way of making a "pasta" dish without including the actual pasta is by using vegetables. This zucchini pasta uses alfredo sauce as well as an abundance of spices to create a truly authentic pasta taste in a recipe that is so much healthier.

Ingredients

- Zucchini (three)
- Butter (one tsp.)
- Garlic (two cloves – chopped)
- Almond milk (one-half cup)
- Heavy cream (one-third cup)
- Nutmeg (one-quarter tsp.)
- Arrowroot powder (one Tbsp.)
- Water (one Tbsp.)
- Parmesan cheese (three-quarter cps.)
- Pepper (one pinch)

Cooking Instructions:

The first step is to make your zucchini into noodles. This can be done with a spiral slicer. Simply use the tool as a grater of sorts on the zucchinis and you will have a pile of stringy, pasta-like vegetables at your disposal.

Retrieve a pan/skillet and melt your butter over a moderate temperature. Once it has heated, add the garlic and let it cook for roughly one minute to the point that it has significantly softened.

Bring the heat down slightly and add the almond milk, heavy cream, and nutmeg. Let this cook at a low temperature.

Get a bowl and throw the arrowroot powder in with the water. Mix these two ingredients until they are consistent and there are no lumps coming from the powder.

Add this to the stove and mix it in. Then mix in the parmesan cheese along with a pinch of pepper for extra flavor.

Whisk all of this so that the cheese begins to meld with the rest of the textures. Leave it heating up to the point that the rest of the sauce starts to become thick with the cheese.

When this has been achieved, take it off of the heat, put it in a platter, and cover it.

Take the zucchini noodles that you have made and put them in the pan that you have just emptied of sauce at a moderate to high temperature.

Cook these for about three minutes to the point that they become softer and closer to the texture of pasta. They will not lose their slight crunch in the middle, however.

Then, put the sauce back into the pan and let everything heat for about a minute while you combine all of the contents.

Remove the pasta and sauce from the stove, put them on a plate, and let everything cool before eating.

Mexican Rice

Rice is an easy and reliable side for any kind of flavors.

While normal rice is far too loaded with carbs, this rice dish consists of cauliflower, as many of our recipes do.

While rice is usually side, and this dish can be too, there are enough vegetables thrown into this to make it filling enough to be a light lunch or dinner rather than just a side.

Ingredients

- Cauliflower florets (three cps.)
- Olive oil (one Tbsp.)
- Garlic (three cloves – minced)
- Jalapeño (one – chopped)
- Onion (one – chopped)
- Tomatoes (two – chopped)
- Cumin (one tsp.)
- Paprika (one-half tsp.)
- Bell pepper (one-half cup – diced)

Cooking Instructions:

Take the cauliflower florets and place them into a food processor.

Put it on a medium setting and only let it go so far that the cauliflower has been broken down into small bits, rather than into one very soft substance.

Remember, the florets should look as much like grains of rice as possible when this process is done.

Get a pan/skillet and put the olive oil in at a moderate temperature. Add the garlic, jalapeño, and onion.

Let these cook for several minutes to the point that the onion has become see-through and the garlic is easy to smell.

Add the tomatoes, cumin, and paprika.

Let all of these cook for several minutes until the tomatoes have become notably soft.

Add the diced peppers and throw the cauliflower rice into the pan now.

Let everything cook together for about three minutes, mixing everything all the while in order to make sure that all of the ingredients and flavors have combined.

When this is done, remove the contents from the stove and put them into a bowl. Let everything cool just a bit and enjoy.

Caesar Salad

A Caesar salad is one of the most common salads there is. While you may often find croutons or unnecessarily fatty dressing along with it, this is a healthy Caesar salad that keeps it simple while also keeping it healthy.

Enjoy this as a standalone meal or as a side to a meat or poultry dish.

Ingredients

Salad:

- Romaine lettuce (one head)
- Shredded cheese (one-half cup)
- Salt (one pinch)
- Pepper (one pinch)
- Cucumber (one-half – chopped)

Dressing:

- Mayonnaise (one-half cup)
- Plain Greek yogurt (one-half cup)
- Garlic powder (one tsp.)
- Grated cheese (one-third cup)
- Salt (one pinch)

- Pepper (one pinch)

Cooking Instructions:

To make the salad, all you have to do is take all of the ingredients from the Salad section and mix them together in a large bowl.

Once those are all combined, you can make the dressing.

To make the dressing, retrieve a bowl and throw in all of the ingredients from the Dressing section.

Whisk all of these ingredients together until they are creamy. Throw the dressing into the bowl with the lettuce and layer everything together.

It is as simple as that!

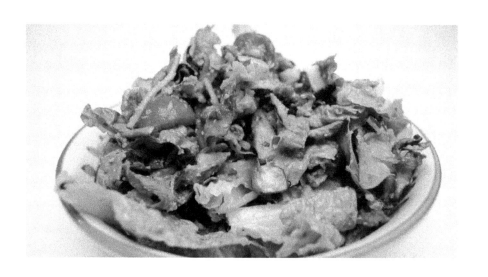

Cobb Salad

Ingredients

- Bacon (three strips)
- Eggs (two)
- Spinach (one cup)
- Tomato (one-half)
- Avocado (one-half)
- Olive oil (one tsp.)
- White vinegar (one-half tsp.)

Cooking Instructions:

The first step in this recipe is to fry your bacon. Do so in the manner that you have in previous recipes in this book.

When the bacon is done, cut it up into bits that can be strewn across the top of the salad. Set the bacon bits aside.

Before you get all your vegetables ready and cut them up to be part of the salad, you can start to boil your eggs.

Put them in a small pot over a stove at the highest possible setting.

Once the water starts boiling, turn the heat off and let the eggs sit for anywhere from six to ten minutes, depending on how hard or soft you want the yolks (the longer you let them sit, the more set the yolks will be).

Meanwhile, you can prepare the veggies. Take the spinach, tomato, and avocado.

Chop the avocado and tomato up into smaller slices and chop the spinach leaves so that they are smaller and easier to eat.

Throw all of these veggies into a large bowl. Take the olive oil and white vinegar and mix them in. Toss everything around until the dressing covers everything.

Finally, take the bacon bits and sprinkle those over the top of the salad.

Then, take your hard-boiled eggs and chop them up into slices. Place them on top of the salad and it is ready to eat!

Cabbage Casserole

Like many of the casseroles and similar dishes in this book, this recipe is incredibly good for you and consists of a simple combination of many ingredients.

This is a meal that can be made heavier by adding about a pound of ground beef, but this version of the dish is vegetarian.

It yields a somewhat large dish so keep the rest for leftovers or serve it for a crowd. Either way, you have a hearty and heavy meal that is perfect as an easy dinner recipe.

Ingredients
- Olive oil (three Tbsps.)
- Onion (one – chopped)
- Bell pepper (one – chopped)
- Garlic (three cloves)
- Diced tomatoes (one can)
- Oregano (one-half tsp.)
- Garlic powder (one-half tsp.)
- Onion powder (one-half tsp.)
- Paprika (one-half tsp.)
- Salt (for seasoning)

- Pepper (for seasoning)
- Green cabbage (one head)
- Shredded cheese (two cps.)

Cooking Instructions:

Take a pan/skillet and put it a moderate to high temperature. Throw in some olive oil to grease it. Once the oil has heated, throw in the chopped onion and bell pepper.

Let this cook until the onion has become see-through and soft, which should take several minutes. Next, throw in the garlic and let it cook for about another minute.

Take the diced tomatoes and pour the contents into the pan, along with the oregano, garlic powder, onion powder, and paprika. Add some salt and pepper for extra flavor.

Take the green cabbage, chop it up into strips and add all of it to the pan.

Cover the pan with a lid and let all of these contents cook at a moderate temperature for about fifteen minutes until everything has become tender and fully cooked.

The final step is to take the shredded cheese and sprinkle it onto the contents of the pan.

Then, cover the pan for several more minutes until all of these have melted.

At this point, move the contents off of the heat, let them cool for several minutes, and take a heaping spoonful.

Feta Salad w/ Pumpkin

One culinary advantage of the keto diet is that many dishes can contain large amounts of cheese.

This salad is no different, as feta cheese is one of the more abundant flavors in the entire dish. As with any salad, this is a particularly easy and convenient recipe.

It is also a very flavorful dish, as the saltiness of the cheese balances very well with the acidity and sweetness of the tomatoes and avocado that are also used.

The yield from this particular recipe is one entrée salad or three small side salads, depending on how you choose to use it.

Ingredients

- Spinach (one cup)
- Roasted pumpkin (one-quarter cup)
- Cherry tomatoes (ten)
- Avocado (one-half)
- Cucumber (one-half)
- Feta cheese (one-half cup)
- Pumpkin seeds (two Tbsps.)
- Kalamata olives (one-quarter cup)

- Olive oil (one Tbsp.)
- Salt (for seasoning)
- Pepper (for seasoning)

Cooking Instructions:

This is probably the easiest recipe in the entire book.

It is as simple as taking your spinach leaves, roasted pumpkin cut into cubes, cherry tomatoes, avocado cut into cubes, cucumber cut into cubes, feta cheese, pumpkin seeds, and kalamata olives and mixing them all together in a large salad bowl.

Separately, mix the olive oil, along with pinches of salt and pepper in another bowl.

Whisk this together until it is consistent.

Then, pour this dressing over the rest of the salad ingredients and make sure they are combined well. Your salad is ready to go!

Fried Eggplant

This a great, unique dish that can serve as a side, a finger-food type appetizer, or a delicious full meal.

The yield of this dish can make it any one of those three outcomes.

Ingredients

- Eggplant (one)
- Salt (for seasoning)
- Almond flour (one-half cup)
- Grated cheese (one-half cup)
- Garlic powder (one tsp.)
- Pepper (for seasoning)
- Butter (one Tbsp.)

Cooking Instructions:

First, take the eggplant and cut it up into slices that are about one-third to a half-inch thick. Put the slices on a plate, add a dash of salt, and let them sit for about a half-hour.

Take a small bowl and break an egg into it. Whisk it up until it is consistent. Take a large bowl and throw together the almond flour, grated cheese (parmesan preferred), garlic powder, and some salt and pepper for seasoning.

Take a pan/skillet and put it over a moderate temperature. Place the butter into the pan and let it melt.

Now, take your eggplant slices and one by one follow this process: dip it in the egg mixture and lightly shake it off so that it does not drip, then dip the eggplant in the almond flour mixture and do the same.

Do this with as many eggplant slices as you can fit into the pan. If you can fit all of them into the pan at once, then all the better.

Let each of the eggplant slices cook in the pan for about three minutes on each side. You will know they are done when they have become brown and crispy, rather than light and soft like how they started.

When the eggplant slices are done frying, place a paper towel down on a large platter and put all of the eggplant there to let them drain. Put the eggplant on a serving platter and enjoy!

Falafel

This dish is falafel only in name. What it really demonstrates is a falafel substitute that is created using, you guessed it, cauliflower.

What you will get from this recipe is eight vegetable-filled patties of this cauliflower falafel. They are on the meal plan as a lunch but can also be used as an appetizer or snack.

Ingredients

- Cauliflower florets (one cup)
- Almonds (one-half cup)
- Cumin (one Tbsp.)
- Coriander (one-half Tbsp.)
- Garlic (one clove – minced)
- Parsley (two Tbsps.)
- Eggs (two)
- Coconut flour (three Tbsps.)
- Olive oil (one Tbsp.)
- Tahini paste (two Tbsps.)
- Lemon juice (one Tbsp.)
- Garlic (one clove – minced)
- Water (three Tbsps.)
- Salt (one pinch)

Cooking Instructions:

Place the cauliflower florets into a food processor as you did with the Mexican rice recipe and pulse them at a medium setting until they have transformed into small bits, rather than into a puree texture.

When this is done, remove the cauliflower from the food processor and put them into a bowl to be used later.

Take the almonds and do the same so that the result is not a full powder but something closer to small bits of almond.

Retrieve a large bowl and put the cauliflower mix and the almond mix together.

Make sure they are well combined and interchangeable. Next, add cumin, coriander, garlic, parsley, eggs, and coconut flour.

Mix all of these together until they have become one consistent texture.

Prepare your stove by adding olive oil to a pan/skillet over a moderate temperature.

While this is heating, gather your mix into separate discs that are about the shape of a hockey puck, though a bit smaller. You should get anywhere from six to ten of these shapes depending on how large or small you have made them.

Next, fry your falafel patties for about four to five minutes per side, or until the outside gets significantly brown.

When all of your patties have been fried, move them to a plate that is lined with paper towels, just like you did for the fried eggplant recipe.

Let the falafel drain here.

Meanwhile, make the sauce that will go on top of the falafel patties. To do this, simply put the tahini paste, lemon juice, garlic, water, and a dash of salt into a blender.

Put it at a moderate setting until everything has mixed and become consistent.

Move your falafel patties to a platter for serving and pour a bit of the sauce on each patty until you have run out. Your vegetable falafel is now ready to serve.

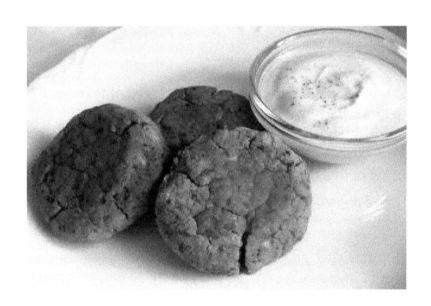

Eggs and Dairy-Free Recipes

Omelet

An omelet presents a good way to get creative with eggs. Since eggs are high in protein and fats, they are a key ingredient for the keto diet, especially when it comes to breakfast.

This recipe makes eggs the lone main ingredients in the omelet.

The trick of this dish is preparing the eggs so that they are fluffy and dense.

Any topping such as hot sauce, cilantro, sour cream, etc. are welcome as an addition to the flavor.

Ingredients
- Eggs (three)
- Water (one Tbsp.)
- Salt (one pinch)
- Coconut oil (two Tbsps.)

Cooking Instructions:

The first step is to retrieve a pan or skillet and get it heated to a moderate to high temperature over the stove.

Separately, take your eggs and break them into a bowl. In this bowl, add the and salt and whisk everything together. Use coconut oil as a non-stick substance.

Add it to your pan/skillet when it is at full temperature.

Next, add your whisked eggs and let them cook. Once the edges of the egg begin to solidify, use a spatula along with a fork/spoon if you need it and fold the egg into a half (omelet-shaped).

When the omelet has cooked through, it can be folded so that it almost resembles a roll or crepe.

At this point, it is ready to serve along with whatever low carb topping you may choose.

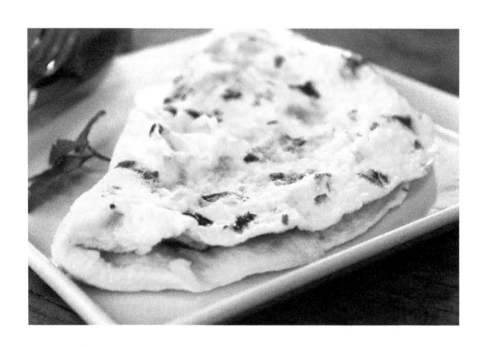

Sausage and Egg Sandwich

This take on the breakfast sandwich exists without bread as the ingredient to bring everything together.

Instead, the eggs themselves are used as bread replacements.

This creates a layered approach to the breakfast sandwich that retains the best and most nutritious parts of the recipe while adding a depth of surprise *and* removing the carbs.

Ingredients

- Butter (one Tbsp.)
- Eggs (two)
- Frozen breakfast sausages (two)
- Mayonnaise (one Tbsp.)
- Avocado (one – sliced)
- Cheese (two slices)

Cooking Instructions:

First, get your butter heating on a pan/skillet. The goal is to melt it to create a non-stick surface for your sandwich ingredients while also adding depth to the flavor.

When the butter has melted, place round molds on the stove. The most common kitchen object that will work for this is the top to a mason jar with the actual seal removed.

Either way, you should have medium-sized round rings that contain an opening through the middle that will work for your eggs.

Take the eggs and crack them, letting them fall into the rings. Then use a utensil to whisk them so that they are consistently yellow, and the yolks are broken.

Cover the stove and let this heat for anywhere from three to five minutes or until they are opaque.

Set the eggs on a plate with one as the top "bun" as it were and one as the bottom. After, set your frozen breakfast sausages either on the stove or in a microwave and heat them through.

Take the mayonnaise and spread it on both of the buns so that you have used a whole Tbsp. and divided it evenly.

Take your sausages off of their heating source when they are done.

Put one sausage on the bottom egg bun and top it with a slice of cheese and a few slices of your avocado.

On the other egg bun, put the other sausage and another slice of cheese.

Then, combine the sandwich so that the layers from top to bottom are egg bun, sausage, slice of cheese, avocado, slice of cheese, sausage, egg bun.

Enjoy!

Egg Wraps

This is another savory breakfast option that centers around eggs and sausage for proteins.

It's a fun and compact dish that you will love, especially if you bring an appetite.

Ingredients

- Eggs (three)
- Salt (one pinch)
- Pepper (one pinch)
- Bacon (two strips)
- Breakfast sausage (one)
- Shredded cheese (one-quarter cup)

Cooking Instructions:

Put a pan/skillet over a moderate temperature. While this is heating, crack your eggs into a bowl and whisk them until they are consistent.

Add salt and pepper for seasoning, and then when the pan/skillet is hot enough, add the eggs. Let the eggs cook until they harden on the outside like an omelet.

Next, take the shredded cheese and add it to the center of the egg. Then, throw in the bacon and breakfast sausage (make sure the sausage is thawed if you are using a frozen one).

Let everything cook until the egg is fully cooked, and the cheese is melted, and the meat fillings are hot.

Carefully remove everything from the heat and fold the egg like you would a burrito. It's as simple as that! Your wrap is ready.

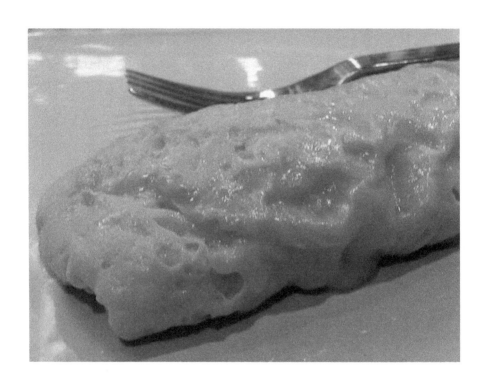

Tofu Stir-Fry

Ingredients

- Extra firm tofu (one twelve-ounce block)
- Sesame oil (one and a half Tbsps.)
- Soy sauce (one-quarter cup)
- Brown sugar (one-quarter cup)
- Garlic sauce (one-half tsp.)
- Peanut butter (two and half Tbsps.)
- Cauliflower florets (one head)
- Garlic (two cloves – minced)
- Red bell pepper (one – diced)

Cooking Instructions:

Take the extra firm tofu and set it between two towels or use one thick towel that is wrapped up.

Once you have completed this step, you should add something weighty to the top of the tofu. One good strategy is to take a small pot and fill it halfway with water.

Set that on top of the wrapped tofu and let it sit for about fifteen minutes. At this point, you should set your oven's heat to four hundred degrees.

When the fifteen minutes are up, take the tofu out from under the weight and out from its wrapping and cut it up into cubes about the size of a normal cube of cheese.

When all of the tofu is cut up, you can put it on a sheet for baking and put in the oven for about twenty-five minutes. You will know the tofu is done when it has browned and shriveled a bit. Let it cool down when it has finished cooking.

The next step is to make the peanut sauce. Take the sesame oil, soy sauce, brown sugar, garlic sauce, and peanut butter (or almond butter if you prefer) and put them in a large bowl for mixing. Whisk all of this well until it is consistent.

Take the tofu from the pan and stir it into the bowl of sauce. The tofu should marinate for at least fifteen minutes as it is imperative that all of the flavor gets absorbed.

Meanwhile, you should start preparing your rice. Take the cauliflower florets and use a food processor to turn them into rice-sized pellets as you have in previous recipes.

When that is done, you can set the cauliflower rice aside.

Get a pan/skillet out and put it over a moderate temperature. Very subtly glaze the pan with some sesame oil or soy sauce and lightly cook the peppers for a few minutes.

When they are done, take them off of the heat, put them on a plate and keep them covered.

Next, you will cook your tofu. Use a slotted spoon to bring your tofu out of the sauce and onto the pan. Once you have all of the tofu in the pan, you can pour a heaping scoop or two of sauce over the tofu.

Cook the contents for several minutes until the tofu has browned. Some sticking is inevitable as the sauce is inherently sticky. As you did with the peppers, take the tofu off of the pan and cover it to keep it warm.

Wash your pan under the sink and scrape any of the remainder of the tofu and sauce off. Then, put it back on the stove at a moderate temperature.

Use a bit of sesame oil or soy sauce again and throw in the cauliflower rice and minced garlic. Let these cook together for anywhere from five to eight minutes.

When they are nearly done, add a bit more of the tofu sauce and mix everything together.

Finally, unite all of the ingredients together in a bowl. Top them with any sauce that is left, and you have a heaping, delicious meal.

Thai Noodle Soup

This Thai soup leans on some of the same flavors as the previous, although it is not nearly as convoluted or time-consuming to put together.

That being said, this is not a side soup. It is full of meat, vegetables, and spices that make this a keto recipe that will keep you feeling full.

Ingredients

- Coconut oil (one-half tsp.)
- Onion (one-half – chopped)
- Jalapeño (one-half – chopped)
- Curry paste (one Tbsp.)
- Garlic (one clove – minced)
- Chicken broth (three cps.)
- Coconut milk (one cup)
- Red pepper (one-half – chopped)
- Chicken breast (one-half pound – chopped)
- Fish sauce (one Tbsp.)
- Lime (one-half)

Cooking Instructions:

Retrieve a saucepan. Take the coconut oil and put it over a moderate temperature to the point that it melts.

When this has been achieved, take your that has been chopped into small slices and heat it for several minutes to the point that it becomes see-through.

Next, mix in the jalapeño pepper that has been chopped up, the curry paste, and minced garlic. Let these cook for another minute to the point that you can smell the garlic.

Then pour in the chicken broth and coconut milk. Whisk all of these ingredients together until they have become completely combined.

Get all of these ingredients boiling and bring the temperature down to moderate once they reach that stage.

At this point, throw in the red pepper. In addition, add the chicken breast that you will also have chopped up beforehand, along with the fish sauce.

Let all of these ingredients cook until the chicken is fully cooked, which should take about five minutes.

At this point, make zucchini noodles as you did in previous recipes by using the spiral slicer.

Do this by using one zucchini. Put the noodles into either one heaping bowl, or two bowls and cover with the rest of the soup.

Take the lime and give one squeeze into the soup for extra flavor. Eat it hot!

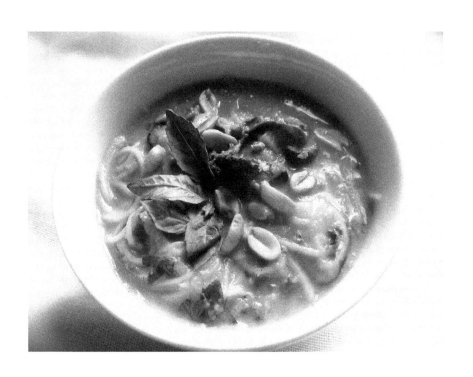

Desserts Recipes

Cheesecake

Ingredients

- Almond flour (one-half cup)
- Shredded coconut (one-quarter cup)
- Butter (one stick – melted)
- Coconut flour (one-half cup)
- Sour cream (one pound)
- Vanilla extract (one Tbsp.)
- Eggs (three)
- Strawberries (one cup – sliced)

Cooking Instructions:

First, set the oven's heat to three hundred fifty degrees. For the crust, grease an eight or nine-inch springform pan, and cover the bottom and sides with foil.

In a bowl mix the almond and coconut flour, shredded coconut, and the butter.

Press the dough onto the bottom and a little way up the sides of the pan.

Put the crust into the fridge while preparing the cheesecake filling.

For the filling, in a bowl, beat the sour cream and softened cream cheese together, then add the vanilla and mix well.

Add each egg one at a time, blending together after each addition. Pour the filling into the crust, spreading it evenly and tapping it on the counter to release any air bubbles.

Place the pan into a deep dish in the middle of the oven and carefully pour boiling water into the dish to come halfway up the sides of the pan.

Bake for one hour to one hour and twenty minutes up to the point that the cheesecake is only slightly jiggling in the center.

Turn the oven off but leave the cheesecake in the oven with the door open slightly to cool for an hour.

Remove the pan from the oven and the water bath and let chill in the fridge for at least five hours or overnight.

Remove from pan and garnish with sliced strawberries or desired fruit before enjoying.

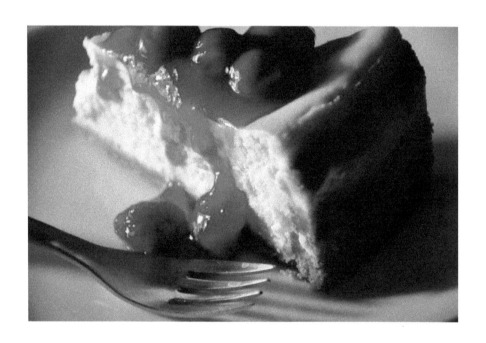

Chocolate Chip Cookies

Chocolate chip cookies are about as classic as it gets when it comes to desserts. Luckily, cookies are a fairly easy thing to make, even when it comes to keeping it up to the keto regimen. These come out soft, sweet, and delicious as ever.

Ingredients

- Eggs (two)
- Butter (one stick – melted)
- Vanilla extract (two tsps.)
- Heavy cream (two tsps.)
- Almond flour (three cps.)
- Granulated sugar (one-quarter cup)
- Dark chocolate chips (three-quarter cps.)
- Keto granulated sugar (three-quarter cps.)

Cooking Instructions:

Set your oven's heat to three hundred fifty degrees. In a bowl whisk together the eggs, butter, heavy cream, and vanilla.

Stir in the almond flour, salt, and keto-friendly sugar and mix well.

Fold the chocolate chips into the batter and form into one-inch balls about three inches apart from each other on a lined baking tray.

Flatten the balls slightly with a glass or measuring cup, spraying with cooking spray if they begin to stick.

Bake the cookies until they are golden brown, which should take around seventeen to nineteen minutes.

Let them cool and serve.

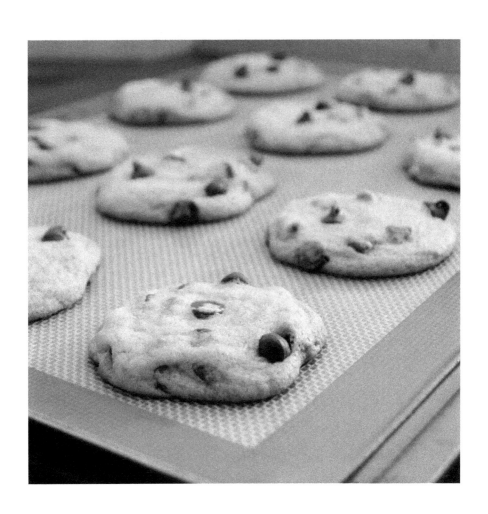

Chocolate Cake

There is not much to say about this dish that the title does not already say. This is a gorgeously soft and delicious chocolate cake that takes little preparation before it bakes.

Ingredients

Cake:

- Almond flour (one and a half cps.)
- Coconut flour (three-quarter cps.)
- Cocoa powder (three-quarter cps.)
- Flaxseed meal (one-quarter cup)
- Baking powder (two tsps.)
- Baking soda (two tsps.)
- Keto granulated sugar (three-quarter cps.)
- Eggs (four)
- Vanilla extract (one tsp.)
- Almond milk (one cup)
- Coffee (one-half cup – brewed)
- Butter (one stick)
- Salt (one tsp.)

Frosting:

- Cream cheese (eight ounces)
- Butter (one stick)

- Cocoa powder (one-half cup)
- Coconut flour (one-half cup)
- Keto powdered sugar (three-quarter cps.)
- Instant coffee powder (one-quarter tsp.)
- Heavy cream (three-quarter cps.)
- Salt (one pinch)

Cooking Instructions:

Set your oven's heat to three hundred fifty degrees and line two eight-inch pans with parchment, then grease with cooking spray.

In a bowl, whisk together the almond and coconut flour, cocoa powder, flaxseed meal, baking powder and baking soda, and salt.

In another bowl, beat the butter and keto-friendly sugar together, using a hand mixer, until the mixture is light and fluffy.

Add the eggs one at a time, mixing well, and then add the vanilla.

Add the dry ingredients and mix until the ingredients are just incorporated, then stir in the milk and coffee.

Divide the batter evenly between the pans. Bake the cakes until a toothpick inserted in the center comes out clean, which should take roughly twenty-five to thirty minutes. Let cool completely before removing from the pans.

To make the frosting, in a bowl beat the cream cheese and butter together, using a hand mixer, until smooth.

Add the keto-friendly powdered sugar, cocoa powder, coconut flour, and instant coffee.

Mix until no lumps remain.

Add the cream and salt and mix until well combined. Place one cake on a cake stand and spread a layer of frosting evenly on top.

Add the second layer of cake and frost the top and sides. It is helpful to do a thin layer of frosting on the top and sides and then chill in the refrigerator for 30 minutes before adding the rest of the frosting to keep the crumbs of the cake from showing on the exterior.

Keep the cake refrigerated until it is ready to serve.

Sauces and Staples Recipes

Guacamole

This dip needs no introduction. It is one of the common favorites to be used for chips or crackers.

You can use this as a topping for a salad or a dip for a fun keto snack recipe.

Ingredients

- Avocado (one)
- Salt (one pinch)
- Pepper (one pinch)
- Cumin (one-quarter tsp.)
- Lime juice (two tsps.)
- Garlic cloves (one – crushed up)
- Paprika (one-eighth of a tsp.)
- Chili powder (one-eighth of a tsp.)
- Scallions (two Tbsps.)
- Cilantro (one Tbsp.)
- Sour cream (one Tbsp.)

Cooking Instructions:

Peel your avocado and take the large seed out of the middle. Scrape the green into a bowl and throw in the lime juice.

Use a fork to mash it up into the proper texture.

Then, simply add everything else and mix it well to the point that everything is combined.

Sweet and Sour Sauce

This is a great dipping sauce. This might go well with the chicken wing recipe from earlier in the book. Otherwise, it is just a great sauce to have on hand when you want to add some sweet flavor to a savory dish.

Ingredients

- Tomato sauce (sugar-free – one-quarter cup)
- Water (one-quarter cup)
- Garlic powder (one tsp.)
- Tamari sauce (one Tbsp.)
- Xanthan gum (one-half tsp.)
- Rice wine vinegar (one-third of a cup)

Cooking Instructions:

Retrieve a saucepan and put every ingredient but the xanthan gum on the stove over a moderate temperature. Mix these contents together and let them heat for about a minute.

Then, add the xanthan gum and let everything simmer. Take a whisk and keep the sauce thoroughly mixed as it heats.

Once the sauce gets thick enough that starts coating the whisk, it is ready to be taken off of the heat.

If you are using it as part of a dish, use it immediately. If it is being used for dipping, you can refrigerate it for now.

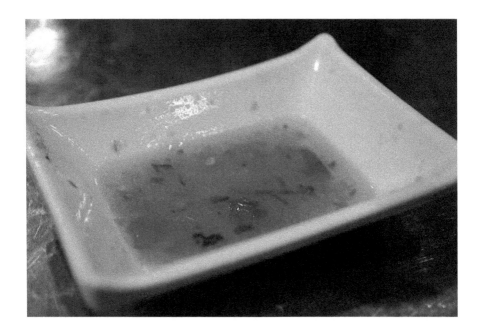

Barbeque Sauce

Barbeque sauce is a great resource to have as it naturally compliments meat and poultry dishes. It could go with any said dishes in this book that you might want to add some kind of sweetness or moisture to.

Ingredients

- Tomato sauce (sugar-free – one large can)
- Apple cider vinegar (four Tbsps.)
- Worcestershire sauce (four Tbsps.)
- Salt (two tsps.)
- Liquid smoke (four tsps.)
- Garlic clove (one – minced)
- Cayenne powder (one-quarter tsp.)
- Onion powder (two tsps.)

Cooking Instructions:

Retrieve a saucepan and put it over a moderate to high temperature. Throw all of the ingredients in, mix them very well, and let it cook at a simmer while mixing.

This should take about five minutes. When it is done, either serve or immediately or jar it and refrigerate it until use.

Conclusion

It is the hope that this book made the ketogenic diet much less intimidating and much easier to understand. These recipes, while low in carbs and conducive to achieving ketosis, look and taste just like the delicious meals that you are used to.

The idea that should get across is that there is really no reason to be hesitant about taking this diet on. Achieving ketosis is as simple as enjoying some delicious, filling meals that happen to be low in carbohydrates.

Other diets focus too hard on stifling eating and creating impractical meals that would never keep a person full.

Through these hundreds of meals that you have just been presented with, it should be clear and evident that the ketogenic diet does not stop you from eating delicious food, but rather encourages you to learn adventurous new meals.

Keto Diet for Beginners Cookbook

From Breakfast to Dessert, Many Tasty Keto Recipes to Reset Your Metabolism, Lose Weight and Improve Your Health without Losing the Pleasure of Food

Audrey Lane

Table of Contents

Introduction

These are concrete recipes that are designed to walk you through the diet, but if you become well-versed in these principles and familiar with the common ingredients, you can be an expert in the ketogenic diet as well.

The important thing to remember from this book is that no meal is impossible to make just because the carb content needs to be decreased.

This book frees you up to enjoy everything from pasta, to meat dishes, to cookies and cake. Ketosis may feel strange for a few days when you get to it, but when it comes to culinary tricks, it is an easy achievement.

Diets are about losing weight, and that is the main promise of this book. If you follow the recipes that have been laid out for you, weight loss will be imminent.

Breakfast Recipes

Crepes

This crepe recipe is also one of the simpler breakfasts you will find in this book. It is lighter than a pancake but contains the same filling and delicious nature.

Ingredients
- Eggs (two)
- Almond meal (one-quarter cup)
- Vanilla extract (one-half tsp.)
- Cinnamon (one-quarter tsp.)
- Coconut oil (one-half tsp.)

Cooking Instructions:

Take the eggs, almond meal, vanilla extract, cinnamon, and coconut oil and put them into a bowl. Whisk everything together like you would a pancake mix then put it to the side.

Retrieve a pan/skillet and put it at a moderate temperature, adding coconut oil for greasing.

Add about one-quarter cup of the batter that you have just made. Turn the pan/skillet in a circular motion so that the crepe covers every end of it.

Cook each side for about two minutes each to the point that they start to solidify and can be removed from the pan with a spatula without difficulty.

Continue to cook like this until the batter is gone which should leave you with anywhere from two to four crepes depending on the size you have made them.

The crepes can be topped with cinnamon or sugar or filled with cream. Just make sure to check the nutrition facts and ensure that the carbs are minimal to absent.

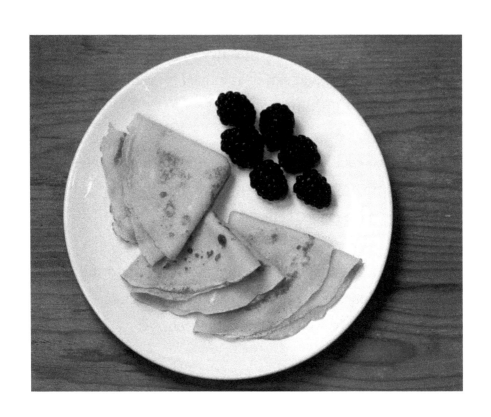

Cheesy Sausage Rolls

These sausage rolls are an abundant and fun breakfast that can fulfill your cravings for food that may be greasier and unhealthier with other ingredients.

This breakfast is shockingly still keto despite the creamy textures and flavor.

Ingredients

- Shredded mozzarella cheese (one cup)
- Cream cheese (one ounce)
- Almond flour (one-half cup)
- Flax meal (one Tbsp.)
- Breakfast sausage (one-quarter pound – precooked)

Cooking Instructions:

First, set the heat to four hundred degrees. Put the shredded mozzarella and cream cheese in a bowl. Then microwave for about two minutes, taking it out every thirty seconds or so to give it a mix.

Then add the almond flour and flax meal. Mix everything together until it becomes doughy. Then remove the dough from the bowl and put it into a cooking pan in a large rectangular shape.

Separately, mix the breakfast sausage with the cheese mixture that you have just made. Once that is mixed, use a spoon to remove the sausage and cheese mix and spread it onto the dough.

Then roll the dough into a large cylindrical shape. Cut this one cylinder in half and place both halves on the pan for cooking.

Let this cook for about twelve minutes up to the point that they have crisped and slightly browned, then they are ready to enjoy!

Banana Muffins

Muffins are a staple of a fun breakfast. In a low carb diet, one can miss fruits and fruity flavors. This muffin helps by providing a banana flavor for this meal.

Ingredients

- Butter (two Tbsps.)
- Eggs (two)
- Coconut milk (one-quarter cup)
- Banana extract (one tsp.)
- Baking powder (one-half tsp.)
- Almond flour (one cup)
- Coconut flour (one-quarter cup)
- Flax meal (one Tbsp.)
- Cinnamon (one pinch)
- Chopped walnuts (one-half cup)

Cooking Instructions:

Set the oven's heat to three hundred fifty degrees. Take a muffin tin and put papers in each space. Take the butter, place it in a bowl, and put it in the microwave for around thirty seconds to completely melt it.

When this has been removed from the microwave, add the eggs, coconut milk, banana extract, and baking powder and mix it together thoroughly.

Next, add almond flour, coconut flour, flax meal, and a touch of cinnamon. Mix everything once more until it is one consistency.

Take the chopped walnuts and throw them into the bowl with the batter. Mix them up with a spoon so that they are evenly distributed across the batter.

Remove the batter from the spoon bit by bit and place it into the muffin holds. Put the tin in the oven for about twenty to twenty-five minutes.

You will know they are done when you stick a knife/toothpick into the muffins and there are no remnants on it when you bring it back up.

Take the muffins out of the oven, let them cool for a few minutes, then scoop one or two out and enjoy!

Cheesecake

Perhaps more than any other dish in this section, it seems impossible for cheesecake to be a keto dish.

This dessert turned healthy breakfast uses almonds as its greatest source of flavor and texture, like many of the other sweet dishes in this book.

You can enjoy anywhere from two to three to stay on schedule with your diet.

This recipe is easier to cook with a greater yield so simply store the rest as leftovers or serve them to a group.

Ingredients
- Almonds (one cup)
- Butter (two Tbsps.)
- Cream cheese (four ounces)
- Cottage cheese (eight ounces)
- Almond extract (one-quarter tsp.)
- Vanilla extract (one-half tsp.)
- Eggs (three)

Cooking Instructions:

Set your oven's heat to three hundred fifty degrees. Put the almonds and butter into a processor.

Mix this up to the point that it becomes doughy. Meanwhile, prepare a muffin tin just like in the last recipe.

Put your dough into the twelve spots for muffins and put in the oven for anywhere from seven to nine minutes.

Put the cream cheese and cottage cheese into the same processor while the dough is in the oven.

You can also add a dash of honey for sweetness. Then add almond extract and vanilla extract, mixing these in.

Finally, crack the eggs into the mixture and blend one final time until the consistency is perfect.
Take this batter and distribute it evenly onto the batter that you have just cooked in the oven.

Return everything to the heat for thirty to forty minutes until the dish reaches the perfect light and soft cheesecake texture. Let cool and enjoy!

Fruit Parfait

This is the rare fruity keto recipe. While most fruits are too high in carbs to be on the keto diet, this dish is an exception.

The presence of strawberries makes carbs about ten percent of this meal. After having this for breakfast, make sure to stay stringent on the keto guidelines.

Ingredients

- Strawberries (one-half cup)
- Water (one Tbsp.)
- Chia seeds (two Tbsps.)

Cooking Instructions:

Take the strawberries and cut them into slices.

Set your stove to a moderate temperature and throw your strawberry slices onto a pan/skillet, along with the water.

Let the fruit heat and melt until very soft.

Next, put the chia seeds, pinches of cinnamon and ground ginger, and a half cup of coconut milk into a small bowl for mixing.

When this is done combining, let it sit for twenty minutes or so.

This will allow all of the ingredients to soak into one another.

When this time is up, add your cooked strawberry as the top layer.

Then, fetch a scoop of Greek yogurt to top everything off. Enjoy!

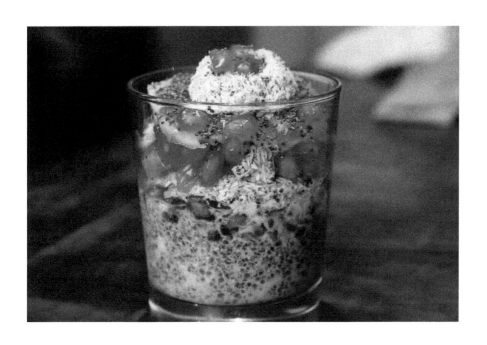

Ham and Cheese Wraps

Similar to the egg wrap, this breakfast presents a good way to condense some of your favorite breakfast flavors into one easy recipe.

Ingredients

- Mozzarella (one-half cup)
- Cream cheese (one Tbsp.)
- Flax meal (two Tbsps.)

Cooking Instructions:

Set your oven's heat to four hundred degrees.

Put the mozzarella and cream cheese in a bowl to microwave for roughly one minute.

When this is melted together and united, add the flax meal. Mix everything up to the point that it is consistent and doughy.

Remove the dough from the bowl and roll it out on a cutting board so that it is flat.

Put some slices of ham and two slices of cheddar cheese in the middle of the dough.

Fold one side over the other and tuck the top and bottom in so that the center is neatly sealed into the dough.

Put your wrap on an oven-safe pan and cook for about fifteen minutes until the dough has become a pleasantly light brown.

Let the wrap cool, cut it into halves and enjoy!

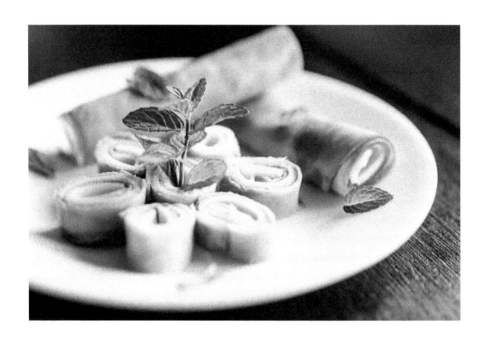

Blueberry Muffins

The final non-smoothie breakfast recipe is a fun and sweet way to enjoy an easy low portion start to the day.

This is another meal that makes twelve muffins so be aware of this yield.

Ingredients

- Lemon (one – for zest and juice)
- Butter (one-quarter cup)
- Eggs (two)
- Almond flour (two cps.)
- Heavy cream (one cup)
- Baking powder (one tsp.)
- Lemon extract (one-half tsp.)
- Blueberries (one-half cup)

Cooking Instructions:

Set the oven's heat to three hundred fifty. Zest the lemon into a bowl and separately melt the butter.

Take the eggs and crack them into a bowl to whisk.

Then, add the butter, lemon zest, almond flour, heavy cream, baking powder, lemon extract, and blueberries.

Mix all of these contents together until they are consistent.

One by one, spoon the batter into a twelve-piece muffin tray. Put this in the oven for about twenty-five minutes.

When they are done, let them cool off and enjoy one or two!

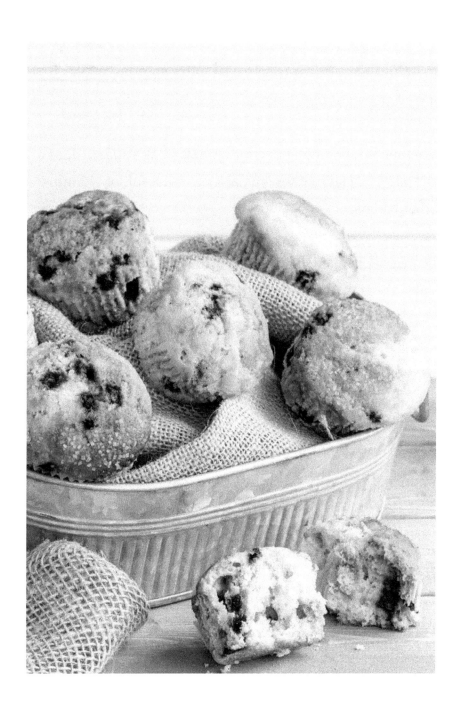

Avocado and Berry Smoothie

Smoothies are a filling way to customize your breakfasts based on your personal preferences.

Whether you're having one for breakfast, as a snack, or as a workout, it's a simple way to pack your diet full of vitamins and nutrients.

The ketogenic diet is all about low to no carbs, which isn't the easiest thing to find with fruit, but berries are notorious for being lower in carbs than most other fruits.

Berries are also very high in fiber, which is an indigestible carb that is great for the health of your digestive system.

Because berries are so low in net carbs, they make a great fruit option on their own, or in this smoothie!

Because these upcoming dishes are not part of the meal plan, the ingredient lists will be provided.

Ingredients
- Water (one cup)
- Frozen blueberries, raspberries, and strawberries (one-half cup - mixed)

- Avocado (one-half)
- Spinach (two cps.)
- Hemp seeds (two Tbsps.)

Cooking Instructions:

Simply add the berries, avocado, and spinach to a blender and turn it on low speed.

Slowly add the water, stopping when the desired consistency is reached.

Add hemp seeds and blend until smooth, or do not blend for added crunch. Enjoy!

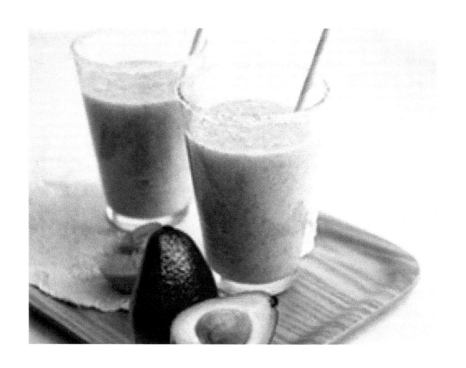

Peanut Butter and Chocolate Smoothie

Creamy peanut butter and unsweetened cocoa powder are the ultimate blend in this rich smoothie.

With under ten grams of net carbs, it is both filling and delicious while sticking to the ketogenic diet.

Peanut butter is also a great source of plant-based protein and quality fats, which will help keep you full for longer.

Ingredients

- One cup of almond milk
- Two Tbsps. of creamy peanut butter
- One Tbsp. of cocoa powder
- One-quarter cup of heavy cream
- One-half cup of ice

Cooking Instructions:

Place the almond milk, heavy cream, peanut butter, and cocoa powder into a blender and turn on low speed.

Begin to add the ice, turning up the blender as needed, until the desired consistency is reached.

Pour your smoothie into a glass and enjoy with a sprinkle of cocoa powder as a garnish.

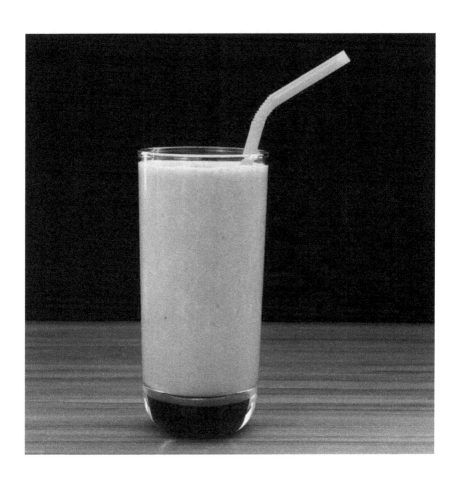

Strawberry and Chia Seed Smoothie

While smoothies are great, they can get a little monotonous if you're using the same ingredients, so to keep things interesting you can switch the typical leafy greens with other low-carb vegetables, like zucchini!

Zucchinis are filled with vitamin c and lots of fiber, and vitamin c is a wonderful nutrient that helps fight cell damage that can lead to heart disease and other ailments.

The chia seeds in this smoothie are also full of healthy fatty acid which is a healthy fat.

Ingredients
- One cup of water
- One-half cup of frozen strawberries
- One cup of zucchini, diced, frozen or fresh
- Three Tbsps. of chia seeds

Cooking Instructions:

Add the strawberries, zucchini and chia seeds to the blender and turn on low speed.

Slowly add the water until the desired consistency is reached.

If you like your smoothie thicker or more chilled then add a few ice cubes and less water

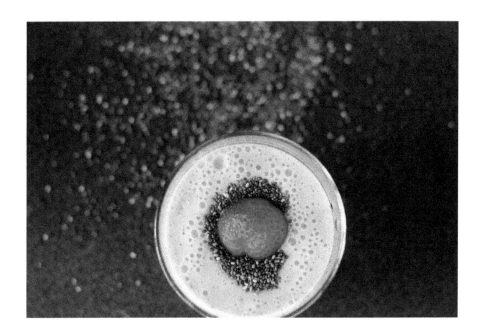

Cucumber and Lemon Smoothie

This smoothie is not only cleansing but has a very advanced water content from the cucumber and lemon which makes this a perfect after workout drink or refreshing snack on a very hot day.

Cucumbers are very low in carbs and very high in water, making them the perfect smoothie as they will make you full and hydrate you, too.

Ingredients

- One-half cup of water
- One-half cup of ice
- One cup of cucumber, sliced
- One cup of leafy greens, such as kale or spinach
- One Tbsp. of lemon juice
- Two Tbsps. of flax seeds, milled

Cooking Instructions:

Throw cucumbers, leafy greens, flax seeds, lemon juice, and ice into a blender and turn on low speed.

Slowly add water, and increase blender speed, until the desired consistency is reached.

Add more ice and less water if you prefer a thicker or colder smoothie. Enjoy!

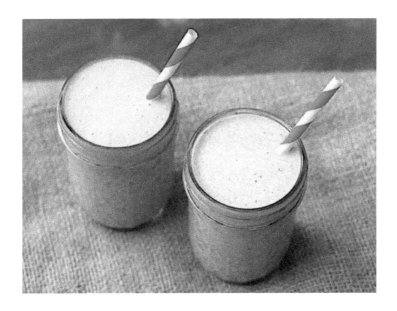

Appetizers and Snacks Recipes

Avocado Chips

Avocados are a dexterous fruit; creamy and full of flavor, great in salads, sauces, or all on their own.

No wonder this avocado chip recipe is so perfect for the ketogenic diet.

While the recipe only uses one avocado, we suggest doing more than that because you will want to always have these chips on hand.

You can easily change the spices in this recipe based on your preferences, but the parmesan cheese and lemon will have you reaching for another chip time after time.

It also may be avocado overkill, but you could easily use these as a vessel for guacamole, however a salsa or onion dip would be our suggestion

Ingredients

- Avocado (one)
- Grated parmesan (one-half cup to three-quarter cps.)
- Lemon juice (two tsps.)
- Garlic powder (one-half tsp.)
- Italian seasoning (one tsp.)

Cooking Instructions:

Set your oven's heat to three hundred twenty-five degrees and line two baking sheets with parchment paper.

In a bowl, mash the avocado until very smooth, then stir in the parmesan cheese, lemon juice, Italian seasoning, garlic powder, and salt and pepper to taste

Place large teaspoon-sized scoops of the avocado mixture on the baking sheet about three inches apart.

With the back of a spoon or measuring cup (sprayed with a little oil if sticking too much), flatten the mixture until the discs are about three inches in diameter and an even thickness so that it will bake evenly and get crispy.

Cook up to the point that the chips are golden and become crisp, they will harden and crisp a bit more while they cool for about thirty minutes.

Let them cool completely and serve at room temperature.

Play around with the size of the chips and the thickness to your liking, but they are best when thin so they will snap like other chips.

Nacho Cheese Chips

It such an easy and crowd-pleasing dish that you are missing out if you don't try it once.

These crisps bake at a very low temperature to get nice and crispy without burning or bubbling everywhere.

Ingredients
- One package of sliced cheddar cheese
- Two tsps. of taco seasoning

Cooking Instructions:

Set your oven's heat to two hundred fifty degrees. Line a baking sheet with parchment paper.

Cut every slice of cheese into nine separate squares, getting them as even as possible so that they bake evenly.

Add the cut cheese to a bowl and add your seasoning, tossing to coat the slices evenly.

Place the slices in one layer, making sure that none are overlapping or touching on the baking sheet.

Bake for about forty minutes, until they are golden and crisp.

They will crisp even more as they cool so be sure not to overbake them.

Leave them to cool for about ten minutes and then remove from the baking sheet and enjoy!

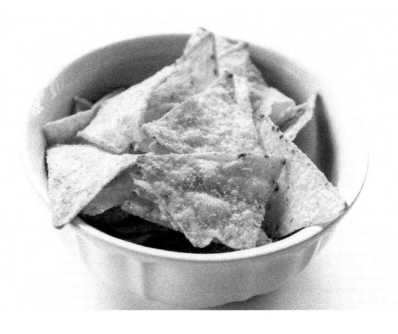

Keto Rosemary Crackers

These crackers are keto because they use coconut flour and almond flour instead of regular flour, and while we use rosemary you could totally use thyme or oregano, or a blend of all three herbs.

These are easy to put together, bake in a short time, and they will store well for up to two weeks.

If you want to preserve them longer than we suggest putting them in the freezer which is a great option if you have a party coming up and want to start your prep well ahead of time.

Ingredients
- Almond flour (two and a half cps.)
- Coconut flour (one-half cup)
- Flaxseed meal (one tsp.)
- Rosemary (one-half tsp.)
- Onion powder (one-half tsp.)
- Eggs (three)
- Olive oil (one tsp.)

Cooking Instructions:

First, set your oven's heat to three hundred twenty-five degrees and line a baking sheet with parchment paper.

In a bowl, mix both the almond and coconut flour together well, and then mix in the flaxseed meal, rosemary, onion powder, and salt.

Add in the eggs and olive oil and combine. Mix well until the dough forms a ball, which will take roughly one to two minutes.

Next, roll the dough to a quarter-inch thickness.

We suggest using parchment paper to keep the dough from sticking to the rolling pin.

Cut the dough into one-inch squares and transfer to the parchment-lined baking sheet.

Let everything cook until it is golden brown, which should take roughly twelve to fifteen minutes.

Remove from the oven and let it completely cool before you eat or store them.

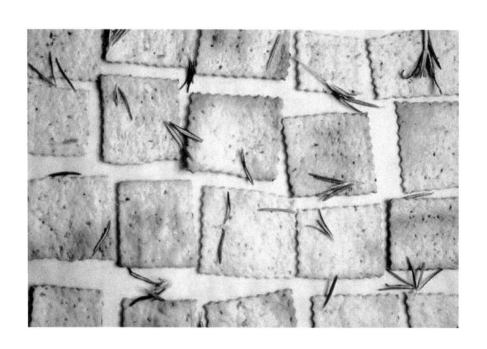

Bacon-Wrapped Asparagus Bites

Anything wrapped in bacon is bound to be delicious, and this recipe is no exception.

This is another great crowd-pleaser for a dinner party, and if asparagus isn't your thing then use green beans or another vegetable you like more.

While only a small piece of asparagus is used in each wrap, definitely go all-in on the vegetables because the cream cheese and bacon may overpower the beautiful flavor of the fresh asparagus otherwise.

Ingredients

- Bacon (six strips, each cut into three small squares)
- Cream cheese (six ounces)
- Garlic (one clove)
- Asparagus spears (nine)

Cooking Instructions:

Set your oven's heat to four hundred degrees and line a baking sheet with parchment paper.

Cook the bacon in a skillet over medium heat until most of the fat is rendered out, but the bacon is still workable (not crisp).

Remove the bacon from the pan and place on a paper towel to drain excess fat.

In a bowl combine the softened cream cheese with the garlic and salt and pepper to taste. Mix until well combined.

On each third of bacon spread about one-half Tbsp. of the cream cheese mixture and then place the blanched and cooled asparagus in the center, rolling the bacon until the ends meet.

Once all the asparagus bites are prepared, place them on the baking sheet and cook for about five minutes until the bacon has crisped and the cream cheese is warmed through.
Do not cook longer as the cream cheese will seep out of the bites.

Serve while warm and garnish with chives or parsley if desired.

Buffalo Chicken Celery Logs

Buffalo wings are ketogenic on their own but serving them for a party appetizer gets rather messy and then there are bones strewn about.

These celery logs are delicious, much less messy, and will be gone so quickly you may not even get one.

Whether you make them for a party or for yourself, you will be left very satisfied and always wanting more, and they are so easy to make that you may as well eat them every day.

Ingredients

- One-third cup of hot sauce
- Two Tbsps. of mayonnaise
- Two cps. of shredded chicken (use a rotisserie chicken for ease)
- Four celery stalks, cut into three-inch segments
- One-third cup of blue cheese, crumbled
- Ranch and chives for garnish

Cooking Instructions:

In a bowl, mix the hot sauce and mayonnaise, then season with salt and pepper to taste.

Add the shredded chicken and mix until well combined. Spoon the chicken mixture in the celery segments.

Sprinkle with blue cheese crumbles, ranch, and chives and enjoy!

Fish and Poultry Recipes

Chicken w/ Mushroom Sauce

This is a very classy and elegant recipe. This time, there are no flashy ingredients to take away from the chicken.

Simply, this dish is designed to center on perfectly cooked chicken and a delicious mushroom sauce that is made to be an exact match for the flavor.

Ingredients

- Chicken thighs (two one-pound thighs)
- Lemon juice (from one-half lemon)
- Salt (two pinches)
- Garlic (one clove)
- Rosemary (one-half tsp.)
- Thyme (one-half tsp.)
- Pepper (two punches)
- Olive oil (two Tbsps.)
- Button mushrooms (one cup – sliced)

- Garlic (one clove)
- Heavy cream (one-half cup)
- Nutmeg (one-half tsp.)
- Parmesan (one-quarter cup)

Cooking Instructions:

First, retrieve the chicken thighs and put them onto paper towels to drain and dry them.

Squeeze the lemon juice onto each of the chicken thighs, in addition to pinches of salt for extra flavor. Let them sit for roughly fifteen minutes so that the chicken can absorb the spices.

Separately, take the garlic, rosemary, thyme, and pepper Layer all of these ingredients onto your chicken.

Next, take a pan/skillet, add half of your olive oil to it and put it over a moderate to high temperature.

Cook both of your chicken thighs in the same fashion that you have cooked chicken in previous recipes (until both sides are browned and the middle is no longer pink).

When this is done, place the chicken on a plate and get going on the mushroom sauce.

To make the mushroom sauce, use the pan/skillet that you had used for the chicken itself, and put the final half of olive oil and sliced button mushrooms in.

Cook them until they significantly soften which should take about three minutes. Add the parsley, rosemary, thyme, and garlic. Cook all of this up for another minute or so.

Pour in the heavy cream and increase the heat to the point that it's simmering.

Then, decrease the heat again and mix everything together until the sauce has become thicker. Add the nutmeg and parmesan.

Let everything melt together, which should take about three to five minutes.

Finally, put your chicken back into the pan/skillet and make sure the sauce completely coats it. Plate a thigh, let it cool to a reasonably warm temperature and enjoy!

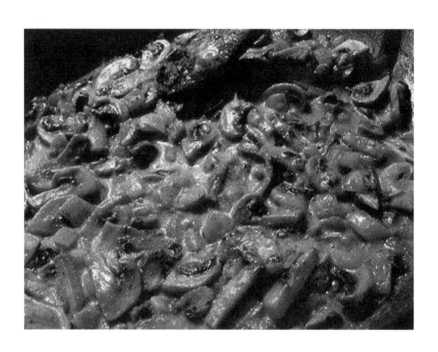

Fried Chicken

When you find yourself in the mood for a fun meal or missing fried foods that you can no longer have on the keto diet, this is the dish for you.

This fried chicken is a dinner in the meal plan because it can be enjoyed with any mix of vegetables such as kale or broccoli. However, it is just as valuable as a snack or appetizer.

Ingredients
- Chicken tenders (eight)
- Dill pickle juice
- Almond flour (three-quarter cps.)
- Salt (one pinch)
- Pepper (one pinch)
- Eggs (two)
- Panko breadcrumbs (one and a half cps.)

Cooking Instructions:

Take the chicken tenders that you have bought from the store. Get a sealable bag and pour all of the juice from a full jar of dill pickles in.

Then, put the chicken tenders in as well, seal the bag up and let it rest for an hour at the very least.

Take a bowl out and throw in the almond flour along with the salt and pepper for extra flavor. In a second bowl, beat the eggs. In a third bowl, put in your panko breadcrumbs.

When the chicken is done marinating, let it rest in each of the bowls in a row, starting with the almond flour, then the eggs, then the panko.

The final step is to fry the chicken. Take a pan/skillet and heaping scoops of fully liquidized coconut oil.

You should pour enough oil into the pan that it overcomes at least one-half of the chicken.

Put the stove up to moderately high temperature and bring the oil to a very high temperature.

If you have a thermometer available, three hundred fifty degrees if the perfect mark for your oil to reach.

Finally, take your chicken tenders and place them in the skillet in order to fry them. Each side should fry for about three minutes.

When they are done, they will have that perfect golden-brown color and bready crunch.

Put them onto a platter along with your choice of dipping sauce.

Chicken Kababs

These chicken kababs are similar to the fried chicken in that they can be a full meal if served with a side of vegetables.

Otherwise, they are a hearty and convenient finger food that are remarkably easy to make.

Not to mention, these kababs are some of the most nutritious meals in this entire book. This recipe yields about six full servings so it is another meal that should be enjoyed with that fact in mind.

Ingredients

- Chicken breast (one and a half pounds)
- Olive oil (one-quarter cup)
- Italian seasoning (one Tbsp.)
- Parsley (one-quarter cup)
- Garlic (four cloves – minced)
- Buttermilk (one-half cup)
- Lemon (for juice and zest)
- Salt (for seasoning)
- Pepper (for seasoning)

Cooking Instructions:

The first step is to clean the chicken and dry it, then cut however much you have into cubes that are about two to three inches.

These will go onto your skewers, so think of each of them as a hearty bite of chicken. When you are done cutting, put them into a sealable bag.

Take a large bowl and throw in the olive oil, Italian seasoning, parsley, garlic, buttermilk, the zest and juice from your lemon, and some salt and pepper for additional seasoning.

Whisk everything together until it is completely mixed, then pour it into the bag with the chicken.

Rustle the bag around so that the marinade is covering every part of the chicken's surface.

Like other recipes, leave the contents alone for at least an hour so that the chicken can absorb the seasoning.

When that time is up, take a pan/skillet and put it on the stove at a moderate to high temperature.

Add some additional olive oil grease the surface. Grill the chicken for anywhere from three to five minutes on both sides until it is browned, and the middle is no longer pink.

Then, retrieve wooden skewers, and place about three bits of chicken on each until you have run out of pieces. A

s written earlier, you can have these kababs with a side salad or any combination of vegetables in addition to a low-carb dipping sauce, of which there are plenty.

Cauliflower Casserole

This meal is included in the seafood and poultry section because it actually contains a notable amount of chicken.

While this time the chicken shares the starring role with the cauliflower, it would be misleading to put this casserole in the veggie section.

This is a very simple dish that you can just throw together if you are pressed for time and it is another one that must be cooked in mass quantities.

Ingredients

- Shredded chicken (one and a half pounds)
- Cauliflower florets (five cps.)
- Buffalo sauce (one-half cup)
- Cream cheese (eight ounces)
- Shredded cheese (eight ounces)

Cooking Instructions:

First, set your oven's heat to three hundred seventy-five degrees. Take shredded chicken that has been pre-cooked. Throw that in a bowl with the cauliflower.

Add buffalo sauce, cream cheese, and half of the shredded cheese of your choosing. Mix all of these ingredients together until they are thick.

Take a dish for the oven that can fit a casserole and spread this entire mixture around into one thick layer.

Then add the remainder of the shredded cheese. Get some tin foil to cover the top of the pan and cook these contents in the oven for around twenty-five minutes.

When that time is up, take the foil off of the top so that the cheese can cook in a more focused fashion.

Cook for ten more minutes or so until the top layer of cheese is fully melted. Remove the casserole from the oven, take out a healthy scoop and enjoy.

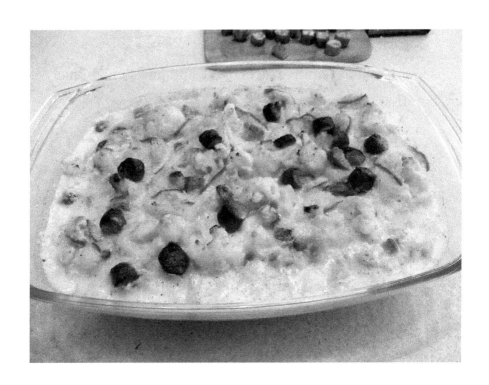

Tuna Salad

This is a lighter dish, and probably more fit for lunchtime as it is indicated on the meal plan.

And while it is a type of salad, it falls into the seafood section for obvious reasons.

This is a dish that requires no cooking and just some minor preparation.

Ingredients
- Tuna (five ounces)
- Mayonnaise (one Tbsp.)
- Cilantro (one Tbsp.)
- Lime (one – for juice)
- Salt (for seasoning)
- Avocado (one – sliced)
- Pico de gallo (one-half cup)

Cooking Instructions:

Take the canned tuna and drain it. Take a bowl and put the mayonnaise, cilantro, and one-half lime's worth of lime juice in with the tuna.

Add a hint of salt and stir everything together until it is thoroughly mixed.

Put an avocado into a bowl then take another half lime and squeeze that juice over the avocado.

Take a fork and press the avocado so that it is very slightly mashed, but still contains solid chunks.

Remove the avocado from the bowl and put it on a small plate. Make a layer of avocado at the bottom that is about two inches in diameter.

Next, take the tuna mixture and add it as a second layer. Finally, take the pico de gallo and add that as the top layer.

Whatever you have not used, you can make it into another serving or you can scramble everything up in one larger salad rather than taking the layer approach.

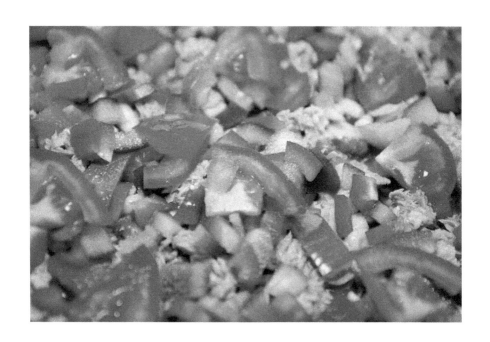

Turkey Skillet

Ingredients

- Onion (one – sliced up)
- Butter (one-third cup)
- Mushrooms (one a half cps. – chopped)
- Garlic (one Tbsp. – minced)
- Chicken base (one tsp.)
- Thyme (one-half tsp.)
- Sage (one-half tsp.)
- Turkey (three cps. – pre-cooked and shredded)
- Nutritional yeast (one-quarter cup)
- Whipping cream (one-third cup)
- Mozzarella cheese (three-quarter cps. – grated)
- Parmesan cheese (three-quarter cps. – grated)

Cooking Instructions:

Set your oven's heat to three hundred fifty degrees. Take a pan/skillet that is safe for the oven and put it on the stove at a relatively high temperature.

Put the butter in first and let it melt to serve as a platform for your other ingredients. Add the onion, the mushrooms, and the chicken paste.

Let all of this cook for twenty minutes or so. It is important to keep them on heat this long in order for the onions and mushrooms to become caramelized.

Next, add the garlic, thyme, sage, and some pepper and stir these in while everything cooks for another minute.

Add the whipping cream and nutritional yeast and continue to cook and stir for anywhere from five to ten minutes.

Then throw in the turkey and half of your parmesan cheese and turn the stove off.

Take your mozzarella and the remainder of the parmesan and sprinkle on top of the mixture you have just made.

Put the pan in the oven and let it cook for anywhere from ten to fifteen minutes.

You will know it is done when the cheese is significantly bubbling and melted.

Remove from the oven, let everything cool for a few minutes, and your mixture is ready to eat.

Meats Recipes

Meatball Sub

When it comes to a meatball sub, what you see is usually what you get.

This recipe, of course, avoids the roll that most subs use as a base. Instead, you will be using cheese as a base for this sub, which makes it even richer, creamier, and more filling.

Ingredients
- Ground beef (one pound)
- Garlic (one clove – minced)
- Basil (one-quarter tsp.)
- Oregano (one-quarter tsp.)
- Pepper (one-quarter tsp.)
- Salt (one-half tsp.)
- Olive oil (two Tbsps.)
- Almond flour (one and a half cps.)
- Baking powder (two Tbsps.)
- Oregano (one-quarter tsp.)
- Cream cheese (one ounce)

- Mozzarella cheese (two cps.)
- Provolone slices (four)
- Tomato sauce (four Tbsps.)

Cooking Instructions:

Set your oven's heat to three hundred seventy-five degrees. The first step is to retrieve a large bowl for mixing.

In this bowl, take your ground beef, garlic, oregano, salt, and pepper and combine them all until they are a moldable.

Once the mixture has reached this texture, take an ice cream scooper like you did for the chicken meatball recipe and form sixteen meatballs.

Take a pan/skillet and add some olive oil. Add all of your meatballs (cook in installments if your pan is not big enough) and let them cook for several minutes on each side until they have browned, and the center has cooked.

The outsides may brown before the center has cooked. If this is the case, then turn the heat down to the lowest possible setting and cook like this until the center has cooked.

Your meatballs are now done. Take them off the heat and plate them for later.

The next step of the meal is to make the cheese dough.

Retrieve two long rolls of parchment paper and a rolling pin.

Get a saucepan and fill it with about an inch and a half of water, then get a bowl that will fit onto the top of the pan so that you can set up a double boiler.

Get the water boiling and then turn the temperature down to the lowest possible setting where it is still simmering.

Take the bowl (which is not over the water yet) and add the almond flour, baking powder, additional salt and oregano. Whisk all these contents together, then break an egg into the mixture.

Then, add cream cheese and mozzarella cheese. Continue to mix everything, though the cheese will not become fully combined quite yet.

Put the bowl over the simmering water.

Stir everything together until the cheese is melted and completely combined with everything else.

You should have a doughy texture to work with.

Turn the bowl over onto one piece of parchment paper, then cover the dough with the other piece.

Use the rolling pin to flatten the dough into a shape that fits into a baking sheet.

Remove the top layer of parchment paper and slide the other layer with the dough on it onto the cooking sheet.
Cut the dough into four quadrants that will hold three to four meatballs each.

Take the sliced provolone and put one into each of the quadrants. Put three to four meatballs into each of these quadrants as well.

Then do the same with the tomato sauce (one Tbsp. per quadrant).
Separate the quadrants (this should be easy as they are already cut.

Use your fingers to pinch the short ends of the rectangles together so that the meatballs are tucked into their rolls.
Then put these in the oven let them cook for anywhere from fifteen to twenty minutes.
You will know they are done when the rolls are nice and brown and crispy and the cheese is fully melted.

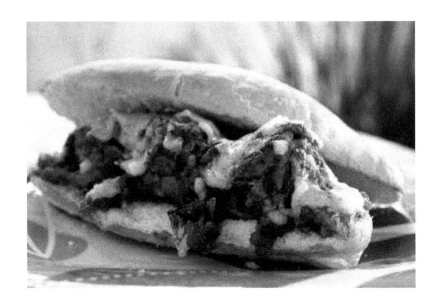

Pork Carnitas

This is another recipe where the meat is used as a wonderful filling for a greater recipe.

These carnitas also use a slow cooker, making the cooking process relatively stress-free, albeit full of ingredients.

Ingredients

- Pork shoulder (two pounds)
- Olive oil (one-half tsp.)
- Cumin (one-half tsp.)
- Paprika (one-half tsp.)
- Oregano (one-half tsp.)
- Brown sugar (one Tbsp.)
- Salt (for seasoning)
- Pepper (for seasoning)
- Garlic (three cloves – minced)
- Onion (one-half – chopped)
- Jalapeño (one-half – chopped)
- Crushed tomatoes (one-half of a fourteen-ounce can)
- Lime juice (from two limes)
- Poblano pepper (one – sliced)

Cooking Instructions:

Take your pork shoulder and make sure it is rinsed and dried. Put the pork in a slow cooker and add olive oil, cumin, paprika, and oregano, as well as the brown sugar, and pinches of salt and pepper for seasoning.

Rub these into the pork so that it can absorb the flavor. Then, throw in the garlic, onion, jalapeño, and crushed tomatoes. Top everything off with lime juice.

Mix all of the contents together then put a top on the slow cooker and let the contents cook on a low setting for about nine hours (you can also cook them at a high setting for about five).

Remove everything from the slow cooker and put in onto a tray for baking. Use a fork to pull the meat apart so that nothing sticks and it is more practical to eat.

Put your oven on broil at a medium setting so that it will be at full heat in several minutes.

Add the poblano pepper to the top of the mixture. Take any liquid that is in the slow cooker and drizzle it on top.

Put the tray in the oven and let it cook for several minutes to the point that everything has become golden and crispy.

Remove the contents from the oven and let them cool down, then take a spatula and give yourself a heaping pile on a plate to enjoy.

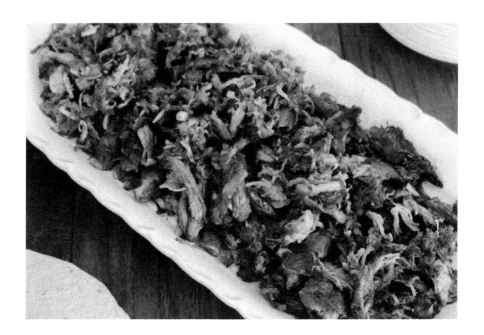

Bacon Salad

While this recipe is technically a salad, the presence of bacon makes it far from vegetarian and savory and rich enough to be an entrée.

There is also an abundance of chicken in this dish. This is probably best enjoyed for lunchtime or as a light dinner.

If you are a fan of bacon, it's a meal that you can make regularly, easily, and often.

Ingredients

- Garlic powder (one Tbsp.)
- Paprika (one-half Tbsp.)
- Parsley (two Tbsps.)
- Chicken breast (two)
- Olive oil (two Tbsps. plus an additional Tbsp.)
- Coconut milk (one-half cup)
- Garlic (two cloves – minced)
- Lemon juice (one Tbsp.)
- Salt (for seasoning)
- Pepper (for seasoning)
- Bacon (four strips)
- Avocado (one – diced)

- Mixed greens (five cps.)

Cooking Instructions

The first step is to set your oven's heat to three hundred fifty degrees. Take a bowl and throw in the garlic powder, paprika, and parsley.

Take your chicken breasts and rub this mixture on each side. Put the olive oil in an oven-safe pan/skillet and then place the chicken inside at a moderate temperature.

Cook the chicken like you have in previous recipes by letting it brown on the outsides. It does not need to cook in the middle as it will go in the oven next. Each side should take around two to three minutes.

Put the pan in the oven and let the chicken cook for about twenty minutes until the middle has fully cooked.

When it is done, remove it from the oven and let it cool for several minutes before you cut both breasts into slices that will fit in a salad.

To make your dressing, put the coconut milk, garlic, the remaining Tbsp. of olive oil, lemon juice, and some salt and pepper into a bowl.

Whisk everything together until it is consistent. Next, fry the bacon as you have in previous recipes. Cut the bacon into strips when it is done.

To put the salad together, put the bacon, chicken, and avocado into a bowl.

Take about the mixed greens and throw them in as well. Mix everything together. You can do this with a salad-mixer or by hand.

Then, add the dressing and repeat. Your salad is ready to serve!

Shepherd's Pie

The final recipe in the meat section is an old favorite. While most shepherd's pies are full of potatoes and bread products, this creatively skirts that by using cauliflower as a substitute.

However, this does not take away from the warmth and richness that a shepherd's pie provides.

This is a great meal for crowds, or if you want to keep leftovers for several days and avoid cooking too often.

This is the only recipe in the section that is not in the meal plan, so the ingredients will be provided.

Ingredients

For the filling:
- Olive oil (one Tbsp.)
- Garlic (two cloves – minced)
- Onion (one – diced)
- Ground beef (one pound)
- Crushed tomatoes (one cup)
- Zucchini (one – diced)

For the topping:

- Cauliflower florets (from one head)
- Heavy cream (one-half cup)
- Shredded cheese (one-half cup)

Cooking Instructions:

Set your oven's heat to three hundred fifty degrees. Put your olive oil into a pan/skillet over a moderate temperature.

When it has heated enough, throw in the onions and garlic and let them cook for several minutes until they are fragrant and soft and clear. Next, throw in the ground beef.

You should heat this until it is significantly browned and fully cooked.

Add the tomato and zucchini and continue to cook everything while mixing for about a minute.

Then put the heat down to the lowest possible setting and let everything cook slowly for about ten more minutes.

At this point, you can remove everything from the heat. Your filling is ready.

To make the topping, take a pot and fill it about halfway with water, then get that water boiling.

Add the cauliflower and boil it for about eight minutes until it is sufficiently soft. When it is done, pour the cauliflower into a strainer and get it as dry as possible.

The dryer it is, the easier it will be to make it into the correct texture for the filling.

Put the cauliflower in a food processor and add the rest of the ingredients from the Filling section of the recipe. Put the processor on a medium setting until everything is smooth and consistent.

To put the shepherd's pie together, retrieve a large dish that is made for a casserole. Put the filling in first, then top it with the topping.

Put the dish in the oven for anywhere from twenty to twenty-five minutes. You will know it is done when the cauliflower topping has begun to brown and it is hot enough to bubble.

When it is done, take it out of the oven and let it cool down for several minutes before taking a scoop.

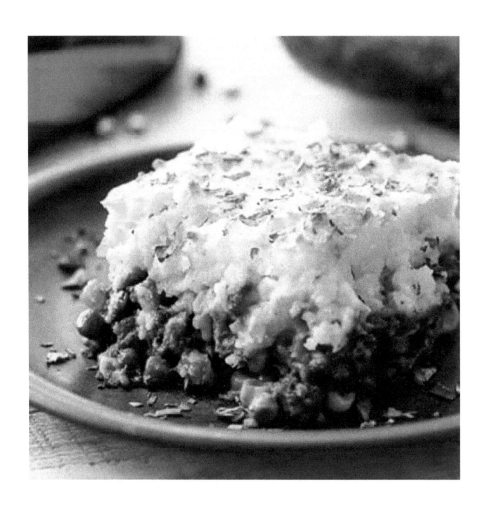

Veggies and Sides Recipes

Roasted Mushrooms

Roasted mushrooms are a great tool to have for the keto diet, because they represent so many options.

You can add them as a side to practically any meal, or you can enjoy them as a quick lunch or snack.

Ingredients
- Olive oil (two Tbsps.)
- Balsamic vinegar (two tsps.)
- Garlic powder (one-half tsp.)
- Parsley (two tsps.)
- Thyme (two tsps.)
- Salt (for seasoning)
- Pepper (for seasoning)
- Portobello mushrooms (one pound – small)

Cooking Instructions:

Set your oven's heat to four hundred degrees. Take the olive oil, balsamic vinegar, garlic powder, parsley thyme, and some salt and pepper and put them all in a bowl. Mix then well until they are combined.

Next, add the small portobello mushrooms that you have cut up into smaller pieces (most likely quarters). Toss everything in the bowl around so that the seasoning coats and covers the mushrooms.

Retrieve a baking sheet that is big enough that you can lay all of the mushrooms out in one single layer. If you do not have one that is big enough then you can use two.

Cook your mushrooms for approximately twenty-five minutes in the oven. You will know they are done when the mushrooms have significantly softened and become the slightest bit shriveled.

Remove them from the oven and let them cool for several minutes. When they are done cooling, move them to a platter for serving and feel free to top them with some extra parsley or a bit of balsamic vinegar.

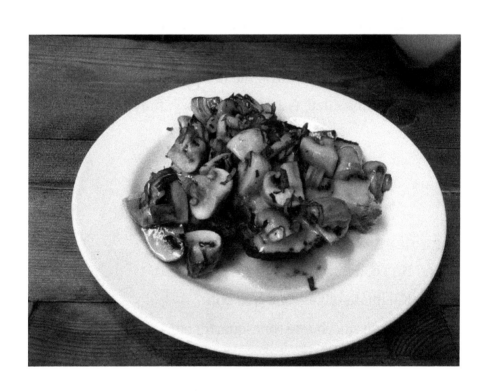

Italian Salad

This dish essentially consists of the ingredients of an Italian sub but in the form of a salad.

The version of it that we have in this book contains pepperoni, making it a side rather than a vegetarian dish.

However, you can easily drop the pepperoni from the recipe and prepare this salad as a quick and easy, fully vegetarian option.

Ingredients

- Broccoli florets (one cup)
- Kalamata olives (one-half cup)
- Mozzarella cheese (one-quarter cup)
- Pepperoni slices (ten)
- Italian seasoning (one small packet)
- Olive oil (two Tbsps.)

Cooking Instructions:

Take the broccoli florets, kalamata olives, mozzarella cheese, and pepperoni slices. Put all of these into a bowl and combine them so that they are evenly distributed.

Get the Italian seasoning and mix it with the olive oil. Whisk these ingredients together until they have combined and are one consistent texture.

Pour your dressing over the salad ingredients in a large bowl and mix everything together so that the dressing is coating the vegetables.

Either serve the salad or immediately, or let it sit, covered in the fridge until you will be serving it.

Vegetarian Noodles

These vegetarian noodles are similar to the zucchini pasta that we used earlier in this section.

However, rather than zucchini, this recipe uses summer squash, carrots, and sweet potatoes as the substitute for the noodles.

Ingredients

- Olive oil (two Tbsps.)
- Summer squash (two)
- Carrot (one)
- Sweet potato (one)
- Red onion (four ounces)
- Bell pepper (six ounces)
- Garlic (three cloves)
- Salt (for seasoning)
- Pepper (for seasoning)

Cooking Instructions:

Set your oven's heat to four hundred degrees. Get a baking sheet and coat it in a light layer of olive oil.

Take the summer squashes and use a spiral slicer like you did for the zucchini, creating noodles out of the vegetable. Then, do the same with the carrot and sweet potato until you have a pile of veggie noodles.

Take the red onion, bell peppers, and garlic cloves and cut everything up into thin slices.

Lay the noodles out on the baking sheet and cover them with a thin layer of the rest of these vegetables that are evenly distributed across the whole pan. Add a bit of salt and pepper to the top of the veggie mixture.

Let this all cook in the oven for about ten minutes. Briefly remove them from the oven to give them a mild toss and mix, then put them back in the oven for another ten minutes (twenty total).

After this time is up, remove everything from the oven and let it cool for several minutes before enjoying.

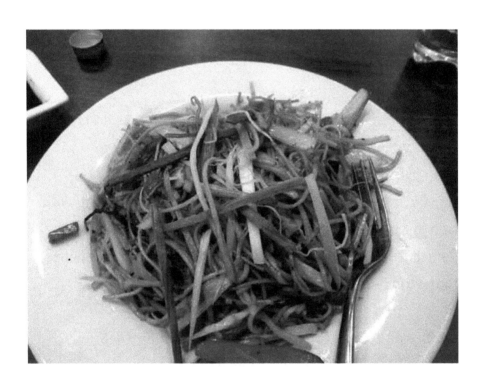

Fried Rice w/ Ginger

This is another rice recipe that uses cauliflower as its base. However, this one goes for more flavor, as ginger plays a major part in the dish.

We recommend that you use this one as a full entrée, as the yield is more than enough for a heaping dish for one person.

Ingredients

- Cauliflower florets (one cup)
- Coconut oil (two Tbsps.)
- Onion (one – sliced)
- Broccoli florets (one cup)
- Carrot sticks (one cup)
- Water (two Tbsps.)
- Grated ginger (two Tbsps.)

Cooking Instructions:

Start by doing what you have done in several of the other cauliflower dishes, which is to put the florets into a food processor and pulse them until they come close to resembling grains of rice. When this is done, put your cauliflower rice in a bowl and set it aside.

Next, get a pan/skillet and add the coconut oil at a moderate temperature. When the pan has gotten hot enough, add the sliced onion and let it cook for several minutes until it has become soft, but not quite see-through as there are other ingredients yet to cook.

Add the broccoli florets, carrot sticks, and water. Put a cover over the pan and let everything steam for several minutes until all of the ingredients, especially the carrots, have significantly softened.

Once you are through this step, take the lid off of the pan and push the contents to one side so that you can add the rice.

Pour the rice in and add the grated ginger. Stir everything and mix it together.

Let everything heat for another five minutes. When that time is up, add a bit of pepper.

Spoon a heaping pile of rice and veggies into a bowl. You may garnish it with a bit of cilantro or scallions.

Broccoli Salad

This is a very fun recipe that turns the word salad on its head. This is about as savory and creamy as a salad can get.

It is remarkably easy to make, and one of the most delicious, unique salads you will have the pleasure of enjoying on the ketogenic diet.

<u>Ingredients</u>

- Mayonnaise (one-half cup)
- Red wine vinegar (two Tbsps.)
- Honey (one-quarter cup)
- Granulated sugar (one Tbsp.)
- Plain Greek yogurt (three-quarter cps.)
- Salt (one pinch)
- Broccoli florets (four cps.)
- Cauliflower florets (four cps.)
- Chopped onions (one-half cup)
- Cheese cubes (one and a quarter cup)

Cooking Instructions:

The first step is to make your dressing. You will do this by putting all of the dressing ingredients into one large bowl for mixing.

These ingredients consist of the mayonnaise, red wine vinegar, honey, granulated sugar, plain Greek yogurt, and salt Once you have all these together in a bowl, simply whisk them until they are combined and consistent.

Cover the bowl with saran wrap and refrigerate it until the rest of the salad is done.

Grab another large bowl for the vegetable portion of this salad. This consists of the broccoli florets, cauliflower florets, chopped onions, and cheese cubes.

Once all of these are together in a bowl, lightly stir the contents so that they are mixed and evenly distributed.

Next, take your dressing out of the refrigerator and gradually add it to the salad bowl. Lightly mix everything around so that the dressing is distributed over all of the salad.

At this point, the salad is ready to serve. Either eat it immediately or cover it and store it in the fridge until you plan to enjoy it.

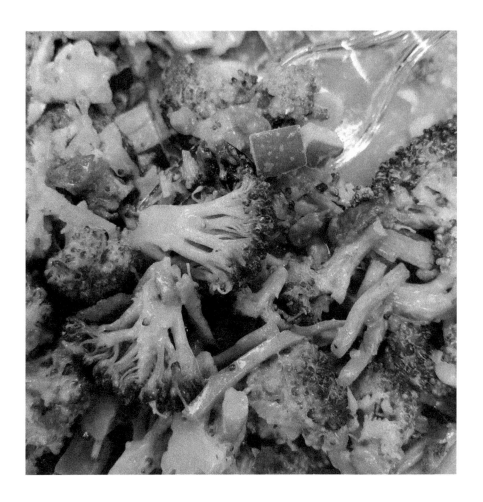

Cauliflower Steak

Ingredients

- Cauliflower (one head)
- Butter (four Tbsps.)
- Roasted garlic seasoning (two Tbsps.)
- Salt (for seasoning)
- Pepper (for seasoning)
- Olive oil (one Tbsp.)
- Shredded parmesan cheese (one-quarter cup)

Cooking Instructions:

Set your oven's heat to four hundred degrees. Take the cauliflower and slice it down the middle evenly three times so that you have four relatively large, abundant slices of cauliflower.

These will act as your "steaks." Take your butter and put it into a bowl. Microwave the butter until it is fully melted.

Then add the roasted garlic seasoning and mix them together so that the liquid and the powder combine to become pasty.

Next, retrieve a brush and lightly apply the butter and seasoning to the cauliflower steaks that you have cut up. Add a bit of salt and pepper to each steak as well.

Take a pan/skillet and add the olive oil to avoid sticking. Put the heat at moderate and throw the steaks on the pan (two at a time or all four if you can fit them).

Let each side cook for about two minutes to the point that they are very lightly browned but be careful not to overcook as they are delicate.

Prepare a baking sheet that is lined with parchment paper. Put the cauliflower steaks onto the sheet and put them in the oven for about fifteen minutes.

Briefly remove the cauliflower from the oven and sprinkle the shredded parmesan cheese onto the tops of the steaks.

Stick the cauliflower back in the oven for anywhere from three to five minutes up to the point that the cauliflower is tender, and the cheese has melted but does not look burnt.

Remove the cauliflower steaks from the oven, let them cool for several minutes and feel free to enjoy all four of them if you have the appetite for it.

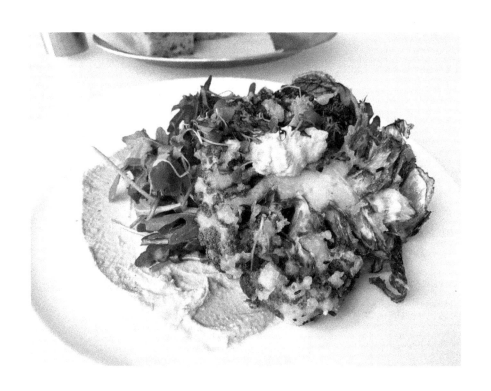

Cabbage Steak

The final recipe in this section follows the same principles as the cauliflower steak recipe above.

It is a dish that is made to simulate a more filling meat recipe while using the consistently healthy and low-fat ingredients.

This dish is slightly more involving because it gets a tad more adventurous by adding some extra flavors to the steak.

<u>Ingredients</u>

- Olive oil (two Tbsps.)
- Cabbage (one head)
- Basil pesto (four ounces)
- Feta crumbles (one-half cup)
- Shredded parmesan cheese (one cup)
- Tomatoes (two – medium-sized)

Cooking Instructions:

Set your oven's heat to four hundred degrees. Prepare a baking sheet for cooking by spreading the olive oil around.

Take the cabbage and slice it into four steaks like you did with the cauliflower head. Place these steaks onto the baking sheet that you have just prepared.

Take the basil pesto and spread it out onto the steaks (one ounce per steak). Next, take the feta crumbles and disperse those over the steaks.

Do the same with the shredded parmesan cheese. Slice up your tomatoes and put those on top of the cabbage steaks as well.

Put the baking sheet into the oven and let everything cook for about twenty minutes until the cabbage has become a bit crispy and the cheese has melted into the steaks.

When you remove the steaks from the oven, put them onto a large platter and make sure you let them cool for about five minutes before eating as the cheese will have made them very hot.

Eggs and Dairy-Free Recipes

Thai Salad

This section gives us one more dish with Thai flavors, and that is the simple and easy Thai salad. There is not much to this recipe other than some greens and some chicken thrown in as an extra source of fat and protein.

Ingredients

- Shredded cabbage (five cps.)
- Shredded chicken breast (three cps. – pre-cooked)
- Scallions (five – sliced)
- Jalapeño (one – sliced)
- Red bell pepper (one – chopped)
- Peanuts (one-half cup – chopped)
- Peanut butter (one-half cup – smooth)
- Water (one-quarter cup)
- Rice vinegar (one-quarter cup)
- Sriracha (one Tbsp.)
- Salt (one pinch)
- Sesame oil (one-quarter cup)

Cooking Instructions:

To make the salad segment of the dish, take the shredded cabbage, shredded pre-cooked chicken, scallions, jalapeño, and red bell pepper that has also been chopped up.

Put all of these ingredients into a large bowl and mix them together. Then add the peanuts that have also been chopped up.

To make the dressing, put the peanut butter, water, rice vinegar, sriracha, and salt into a bowl. Microwave this bowl until the peanut butter has become soft enough to be mixed around.

When the microwaving is done, add your sesame oil. Whisk everything thoroughly until the dressing is consistent.

Next, simply pour the dressing over the salad ingredients and mix everything so that the dressing coats all of the ingredients. Enjoy!

Lemon Chicken Wings

A bonus addition to our poultry and seafood section, these chicken wings are a fun and fairly simple meal to throw together for parties or for a quick, meaty fix. This, as well as the three following recipes are not on the meal plan so the ingredients will be provided.

Ingredients

- Chicken wings (about three pounds)
- Avocado oil (two Tbsps.)
- Lemon juice (one-half cup)
- Salt (for seasoning)
- Pepper (for seasoning

Cooking Instructions:

Take a large, sealable plastic bag and throw all of the ingredients in there together. Make sure the bag is sealed, then gently move the bag around so that all of the liquid coats the chicken.

The wings should marinate for at least four hours, or overnight to make it easier.

When marinating is coming to an end, set your oven's heat to four hundred twenty-five degrees.

Line a baking sheet with aluminum foil and take the chicken wings out of the bag. Let them cook until the wings are done.

You will know to take them out when the skin has become golden brown and the middle no longer holds any pink you stick a fork in to check.

This should take about a half an hour.

Take the wings out of the oven, let them cool down, and then eat hot.

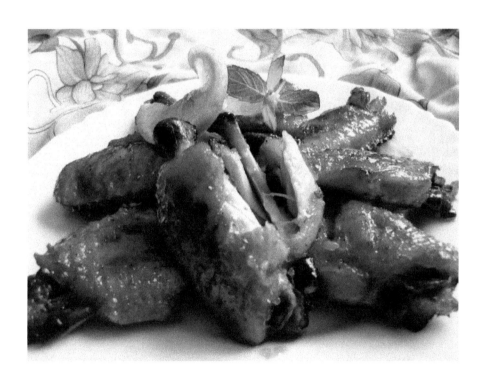

Salmon Bites

Like the chicken wings, these salmon bites are a fun dish that you can put together if you want a snack that you can produce in bulk, or a meal that contains some extra protein.

Ingredients

Bites:

- Canned salmon (twenty-four ounces)
- Pork rinds (three-quarter cps.)
- Eggs (five)
- Mayonnaise (one-quarter cup)
- Jalapeño pepper (one-half – chopped up)
- Dried dill (one-half tsp.)
- Garlic powder (three-quarter tsps.)
- Red pepper flakes (one-eighth of a tsp.)
- Salt (for seasoning)
- Pepper (for seasoning)
- Avocado oil (one Tbsp.)

Sauce:

- Mayonnaise (one-quarter cup plus an additional two Tbsps.)
- Mustard (one Tbsp.)

- Lemon juice (one Tbsp.)
- Dried dill (two tsps.)
- Apple cider vinegar (one Tbsp.)
- Lemon zest (from one lemon)
- Garlic powder (one-quarter tsp.)

Cooking Instructions:

Take all of the ingredients for the bites, besides the avocado oil and throw them into one large bowl for mixing. Combine them thoroughly using an electric whisk.

When the mixture has become consistent and malleable, use your hands to make twenty-four small balls of salmon. Put them on a plate and slightly flatten them.

Take a pan/skillet and put it over a moderate temperature. Add the avocado oil, then fry each of the salmon bites, cooking as many as you can at one time.

Each side needs about four to six minutes to get golden brown and fully cooked. Once you are done cooking all of the salmon bites, set them aside on a platter.

For the sauce, take all of the ingredients that are listed in the Sauce section and put them in a medium-sized bowl.

Use a whisk to combine everything.

That is all there is to it! Put your sauce in a dipping bowl and you can serve your salmon bites, dipping them into the sauce every time you eat one.

Stuffing

This is yet another culinary favorite that is usually associated with carbs.

But we give this stuffing another keto spin by using nuts and dense vegetables to achieve the same kind of hearty and full texture that a normal stuffing has.

Ingredients

- Pumpkin seeds (two Tbsps.)
- Garlic (one Tbsp. – minced)
- Coconut oil (three Tbsps.)
- Yellow onion (one – chopped)
- Celery (six ounces – chopped)
- Cauliflower florets (one head)
- Chicken broth (one-quarter cup)
- Mushrooms (eight ounces – chopped)
- Rosemary (two Tbsps.)
- Sage (one Tbsp.)
- Salt (for seasoning)
- Pepper (for seasoning)

Cooking Instructions:

Get a pan/skillet and put it over a moderate temperature. Add the coconut oil and, once it melts, add the pumpkin seeds and let those cook for a few minutes until they become golden.

Then, add the garlic and let that cook for another two or so minutes to the point that you can smell it well.

Bring the heat up and add the onion and celery. Let these cook for about eight minutes to the point that they are soft. At this point, you can add the rest of the ingredients.

Mix everything up it is combined and continue to gently stir intermittently as everything cooks. This process should take about a half an hour.

You will know that these ingredients are done cooking when they have significantly softened and are starting to come apart.

Remove everything from the heat, place into a large bowl, and take a heaping scoop to enjoy. Cover and refrigerate whatever you do not eat.

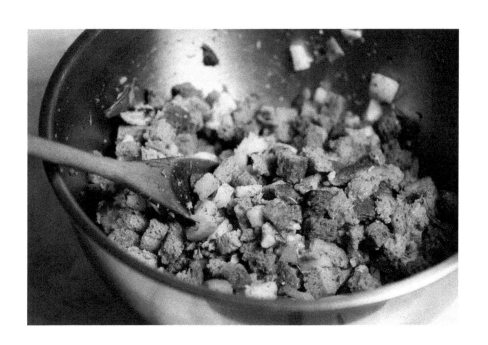

Coffee Cake

The final recipe in this section is a perfect transition into our next section which consists entirely of desserts.

This coffee cake is miraculously keto. It can be a dessert, a breakfast, or a snack for any time of day.

Ingredients

Cake:

- Eggs (nine)
- Coconut flour (two thirds of a cup)
- Coconut oil (two thirds of a cup)
- Cream of tartar (two tsps.)
- Vanilla extract (two tsps.)
- Cinnamon (one-half tsp.)
- Baking soda (one tsp.)

Crumble:

- Shredded coconut (one cup plus an additional three Tbsps.)
- Coconut flour (three Tbsps.)
- Coconut oil (five Tbsps.)
- Cinnamon (one and one-quarter tsp.)

Cooking Instructions:

Set your oven's heat to three hundred fifty degrees. Get a deep square baking pan and grease it with a bit of canola oil.

Take your eggs and use an electric mixer to whisk them until they are thick, which should take about two minutes.

Add the vanilla extract and coconut oil at this point and continue to mix until they are completely combined with the eggs.

Take a bowl and add the coconut flour and baking soda. Mix them together until they are combined.

Take this bowl and gradually add it to the egg mixture with the electric mixer still going at a low setting. After a while, the mixture will form into a doughy texture.

When the dough is finished, put it into the baking pan and throw that in the oven. That should cook for around thirty-five minutes.

While the structure of the coffee cake is cooking, you can put together the crumble that goes on top of the cake.

Add all of the ingredients from the Crumble section into one bowl. Mix everything fairly strongly so that it is really all whisked together.

When the coffee cake is done cooking, take it out of the oven and immediately spread the crumble on top of it.

Once everything has cooled enough, cut a slice out and enjoy the cake hot. Cover whatever you do not eat.

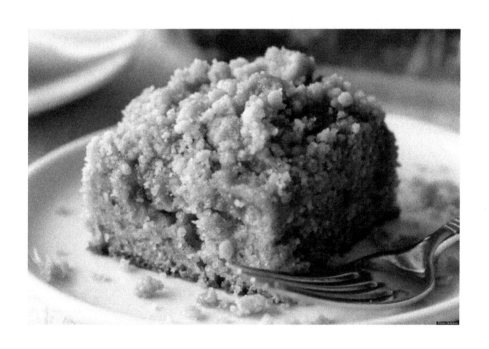

Desserts Recipes

Chocolate Frozen Cream

This is as close to ice cream as you can get on the ketogenic diet. It is designed to be a bit creamier than ice cream, but it delivers the same kind of sweetness and wonderful texture.

Ingredients

- Heavy cream (one cup)
- Cocoa powder (two Tbsps.)
- Vanilla extract (one tsp.)
- Almond butter (one tsp.)
- Liquid stevia (five drops)

Cooking Instructions:

Put the heavy cream into a bowl for mixing. Use a whisk and beat it for a few minutes until it is creamier and somewhat firm.

Next, you can throw in the rest of the ingredients and continue to whisk. Using a whisk by hand should be sufficient, but if you find that it is not getting creamy enough or you are getting too tired, you can use an electric mixer.

Once the mixture has achieved the creamy consistency that it is supposed to (think whipped cream), move it into a bowl. Once the mixture is in that bowl, place it in the freezer.

It should take about thirty minutes for the cream to get cold enough to reach the correct texture. At this point, take it out of the freezer and enjoy immediately!

Peanut Butter Bars

This is an absolutely scrumptious dessert that does not require any baking whatsoever. These brownie-like bars are perfect for anyone with a sweet tooth which needs that chocolatey fix. This is a personal favorite recipe that is perfect for anyone who is in need of a unique new dessert.

Ingredients

Peanut Butter Layer:
- Peanut butter (one cup – smooth)
- Keto granulated sugar (one Tbsp.)
- Coconut flour (two-thirds of a cup)

Chocolate Layer
- Peanut butter (two Tbsps. – smooth)
- Coconut oil (four Tbsps.)
- Keto granulated sugar (two Tbsps.)
- Cocoa powder (one-third of a cup)

Cooking Instructions:

Take out a bowl for mixing and throw in all of the ingredients from the PB Layer section. Lightly mix everything together with a spatula or a large spoon.

At this point, you should use your hands to toss everything together in a sort of kneading technique. Then everything will begin to feel doughy.

Once you have made these contents into a dough, you should transfer it to a brownie pan that has been covered with parchment paper.

Once you have the dough in the pan, press down on it so that it reaches every edge. Use a spatula to smooth the layer. Then, put the pan in the freezer.

Take out another bowl for mixing and throw in the peanut butter and coconut oil from the Choc. Layer section.

Put them in the microwave for about thirty seconds to melt them to the right texture. When that is done, mix them together to make them consistent.

At this point, take the keto sugar and cocoa powder and add it to the melted mixture.

Whisk these ingredients fairly aggressively to make sure that all of the textures unite.

Then, you can take the peanut butter layer out of the freezer and pour the chocolate layer on top of it.

Since the peanut butter will be chilled, you should spread the chocolate around the top quickly and then pop the pan back into the freezer.

Let this pan sit in the freezer for about a half an hour.

When that time is up, take it out and prepare to cut them into squares. To do this, run your knife under hot water.

This will allow it to break through the hard layer of chocolate. Cut everything up into squares or rectangles of your preference and enjoy.

Store any that you do not eat in the refrigerator.

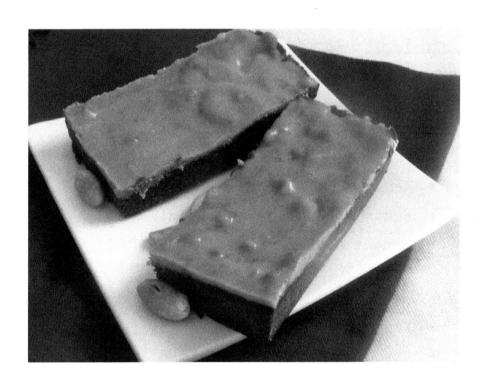

Lemon Squares

This is another dessert dish that comes together to create several squares of finger food. Although the centerpiece of this recipe is lemon, it still presents a sweet and refreshing dessert option for those who want to ere away from chocolate.

Ingredients

Crust:
- Almond flour (one cup)
- Coconut flour (one-quarter cup)
- Keto granulated sugar (one-quarter cup)
- Butter (three Tbsps. – melted down)
- Lemon zest (from one-half lemon)

Filling:
- Keto granulated sugar (three-quarters of a cup)
- Almond milk (one-half cup)
- Butter (one Tbsp. – melted down)
- Lemon juice (one cup)
- Lemon zest (from one-half lemon
- Eggs (five – beaten)

Topping:

- Almond flour (two Tbsps.)
- Coconut chips (three-quarter cps.)
- Butter (one-half Tbsp.)

Cooking Instructions:

Set your oven's heat to three hundred fifty degrees. Get a square brownie pan prepared with some non-stick spray.

Take a bowl for mixing and add all of the Crust ingredients but the butter. Stir them all together until they are combined in texture.

Then add the butter and stir it around with a spoon, maybe even your hands, to make sure it melds with the flours.

When the texture has become dough-like, take it out of the bowl and press it into the bottom of the pan that you have prepared.

Put it in the oven and let it cook for about fifteen minutes. Remove the dough from the oven and let it cool while you make the filling.

To make the filling, get a saucepan, put it over a moderate temperature and add the keto sugar, butter, lemon zest, and almond milk. Stir while these ingredients heat.

Once the butter and sugar has completely liquified, add the lemon juice. Next, whisk the eggs in and keep stirring so that everything blends together. Cooking all of this should take another eight or so minutes.

Dump the filling onto the crust that has been sitting to the side. Put these contents in the oven for another fifteen or so minutes.

While this is cooking, get going on the topping. Take all of the ingredients from the Topping section and put them into a processor.

Set it to moderate and let these ingredients pulse until they are grainy, but not too soft.

Take the pan out of the oven when it is ready and add you topping to the top layer. Then, return it to the oven for five more minutes.

When you take it out of the oven, let it cool down for several minutes, then cut out squares or rectangles just like you did in the last recipe.

Your lemon squares are ready to eat, and you can keep your leftovers refrigerated and covered.

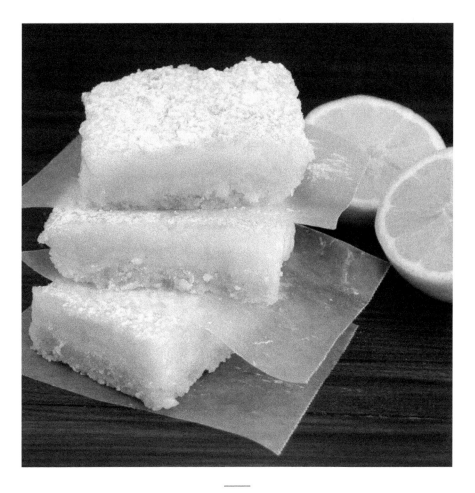

Sauces and Staples Recipes

Tapenade

Tapenade is a sophisticated staple that can be used as a dip for crackers, or even as a topping on things like meat and poultry.

Ingredients

- Kalamata olives (about ten ounces)
- Thyme (one Tbsp.)
- Parmesan cheese (one ounce)
- Olive oil (one-quarter cup)
- Garlic cloves (two)
- Lemon juice (one tsp.)
- Salt (one pinch)
- Pepper (one pinch)

Cooking Instructions:

Take your olives, draining and rinsing them in the sink. Set them on a paper towel to dry.

When they are done drying, put them in a food processor along with the thyme, parmesan, and garlic. Blend it on a high setting until it is pasty.

Then, throw the olive oil and lemon juice in and blend at a low setting for five minutes so that everything completely unites.

If necessary, take a spoon and scrape the sides every couple minutes.

Put the salt and pepper in and blend everything for another two minutes.

Place the tapenade into a bowl and refrigerate it until serving, ensuring that it is covered.

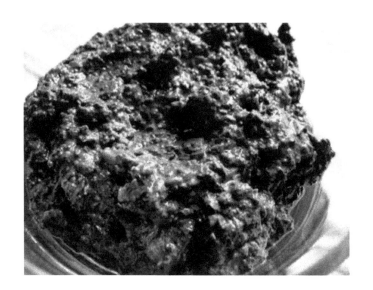

Enchilada Sauce

The final recipe in this section sticks to its name.

It is a great sauce to add to dishes such as burritos, enchiladas, or Mexican rice.

Ingredients

- Cayenne (one-quarter tsp.)
- Oregano (two tsps.)
- Cumin (three tsps.)
- Onion powder (two tsps.)
- Tomato puree (twelve ounces)
- Coriander (two tsps.)
- Butter (three ounces)
- Salt (one-half tsp.)
- Pepper (one-half tsp.)

Cooking Instructions:

Retrieve a saucepan, put it over a moderate temperature, and add the butter. Let the butter melt, then add everything but the tomato puree.

Let these ingredients cook for a few minutes until you can smell them. Then, add the puree and make sure to stir it in very well.

Let everything heat at a simmer for about five minutes. Like the other sauces, either use it immediately, or store it covered in the fridge.

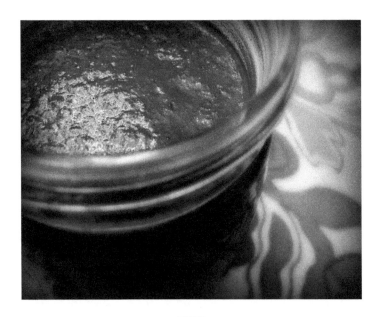

Conclusion

For the past ten years or so, no diet has been as widespread in its usefulness and popularity as the keto diet. Everyone from nutritionists to professional basketball stars have come out in support of its massively effective results for losing weight and improving general nutritional health.

Most people who struggle with weight problems and all of the health drawbacks that come with it usually fall victim to the fundamental imbalances in the normal everyday diet that is advertised in mass media.

Everything from chips, to bread, to pizza, to burgers and fries contain high volumes of fat and carbohydrates that make losing wait an impossibility and make being healthy even harder.

Lightning Source UK Ltd.
Milton Keynes UK
UKHW020903220321
380765UK00001B/75